NCO: No Compassion Observed

Life with Lyme Disease in the Military

By
Sue Vogan

Lyme Disease Books and Resources
www.LymeBook.com

BioMed Publishing Group

ISBN 10: 0-9763797-3-2.
ISBN 13: 978-0-9763797-3-7.
Copyright © 2007 by Sue Vogan

BioMed Publishing Group
P.O. Box 9012
South Lake Tahoe, CA 96158
www.LymeBookStore.com

Lyme Disease books, videos & resources: www.LymeBookStore.com

Disclaimer

The author is not a physician or doctor, and this book is not intended as medical advice. It is also not intended to prevent, diagnose, treat or cure disease. Instead, the book is intended only to share the author's research, as would an investigative journalist. The book is provided for informational and educational purposes only, not as treatment instructions for any disease.

Dedication

I dedicate this book to Linda, for without her faith and support, I might never have found the strength to tell this story.

Foreword

On my first visit to a Marine Corps Exchange I rummaged through the racks of t-shirts, looking for the quintessential shirt for a new 2nd Lieutenant, and saw a rack filled with shirts with sayings like "Marine Wife – the hardest job in the Corps" and similar odd-seeming statements.

Over the course of my 20-plus years as an Officer of Marines and, for the past 8, as a Civilian Defense Counsel working aboard bases for all services, worldwide, I've learned the universal applicability of that shirt's slogan to all branches of our Armed Forces.

I first encountered Sue Vogan during my representation of Army SGT Mark Walker, the Army Engineer accused of negligent homicide in connection with the accidental killing of two South Korean teen girls in June of 2002, near Camp Casey and the DMZ.

As in the case of so many servicemen accused of horrible offenses, I found that SGT Walker's chain-of-command had written him off as lost and that he was ostracized by his superiors, merely because he was charged with a terrible offense and because he was the subject of heated and oft-times violent protests by the Korean citizens nearby and in Seoul.

It was at this time that Sue Vogan contacted me, explained that her husband had been stationed at Camp Casey, and offered to assist the Walker family in fund-raising efforts in order for them to pay my fees.

It was only after SGT Walker's acquittal at a General

Court-Martial on all charges that his chain-of-command again assumed its position of support for him and resumed treating him like any other soldier.

Sue and I had never met – in fact, we still haven't – but I came to know her to be a strong-willed military spouse, resolute in support of her husband in his career and caring for the plight of other servicemen and their families.

Sue has proven to be a tireless advocate for military families – a fundamental part of our greatest national asset, our troops.

This book by Sue presents but a brief snapshot of the experiences of this remarkable and dedicated woman, and is a valuable reference for military families and for those officers and senior enlisted personnel who would endeavor to lead our forces and who must also ensure the tranquility of the military family.

To Sue and her family: as we say in the Naval Service, "Fair winds and following seas," and semper fidelis.

Guy Womack
LtCol, USMC(Ret)

Table of Contents

Acknowledgments

Acknowledgements: To my editor, Joyce Fowler, for being as patient as anyone could ever be, and to the U.S. Army for making me see that no one could take everything away from me; and to my mother, who taught me what a sense of humor and determination was long before I actually needed them.

CHAPTER I

The Military Lifestyle

My association with the U.S. Army started in 1996 when I met and married Tim. He was a seasoned Staff Sergeant and a by-the-book soldier. While he was intimidating in his uniform, he had a way with soldiers that most Non Commissioned Officers would like to have learned. Tim got the job done, and he never made enemies along the way.

Like most enlisted military wives, I held a full time job and chose to volunteer for just about every organization affiliated with the military. I organized Family Readiness Groups, taught Army Family Team Building, and even branched out to the local community with various projects. Unlike most military wives, my association would be bumpy.

Outside the main gate at Ft. Sill, Oklahoma, the business establishments stand steadfast to serve our soldiers. If you are interested in a little spank and tickle, there are plenty of massage parlors dotted along the route into the gate that will provide this service. There are also pawn shops, lemon car lots, check cashing joints that will accept post dated checks for a large fee, quick loan enterprises, strip clubs, bars, and cheap fast food restaurants. This sight is not uncommon outside the guarded gates of many military installations all over the United States.

Long lines of vehicles always wait to pass through the checkpoint. Once inside the gates, the civilian law officers are replaced by the Military Police. Signs that stand like wooden soldiers along the sides of the paved roads direct visitors to everything from the Commissary (military grocery story) to the American Red Cross Office. The hospital is centrally located, and it looms above every other building on the post. There is a PX (Post Exchange -- the military's version of a department store), a Class Six (liquor store), a lawn and garden shop also stocked with toys, and a cleaner for BDU's (Battle Dress Uniforms). The military post is a self-contained environment. If one were stranded within this fenced-in compound that stretched for miles in all directions, they would have no worries about their survival. Food, clothing, shelter, healthcare, churches, gasoline, banking, and even a car wash would provide them with the comforts seen in the civilian world.

Within the installation, you are transported into another land. This is the world of the shrubs (soldiers in camouflage) and brass, where nothing is as it appears. There is no rule or regulation that cannot be bent or broken should it serve those in command. The fairness or justice of the civilian world is not to be found here. Whether right or wrong, the only way is the military way. A visitor would never realize that the command could force a soldier to protect the post under an "orange" alert, and yet provide no ammunition for his weapon. Who would suspect that the soldiers are unsafe while attending a training exercise without sleep for two or three days? No one on the outside would know! Soldiers only complain among themselves, because to do otherwise would be grounds for punishment. No soldier wants to scrub floors or sweep up after pulling a 24-hour duty as CQ (Charge of Quarters). It's better to keep their lips tightly sealed. This is the way of the U.S. Army, and however long you are a soldier or family member, it is the ONLY way. Right or wrong. Welcome to our world.

The wives face a similar challenge. The PX is designed for officers' wives. The clothes for sale are geared for functions only officer's wives attend, and there is nothing much above a size 12 hanging on the racks. The wives of enlisted soldiers learn not to complain. It wouldn't change anything, because this is the way it has always been done. Wives wouldn't dare complain. They have learned that their husbands would have to pay for their actions. Shopping in town at the local Wal-Mart was the only other option, and it was always jam packed on paydays. Just think of how much money could be made by the military if they stocked a line for en-listed wives!

I knew how the enlisted wives felt. I was one of them, and I spent a lot of time as a volunteer for Army Family Team Building (AFTB). It was there that I taught the new wives what the U.S. Army wanted them to know. Most of the classes consisted of common sense information. The women learned how to sign up for volunteer positions and were told about Family Support Groups (FSG was changed shortly after 1996 to Family Readiness Groups or FRG). Some of the topics were idealistic nonsense the U.S. Army was try-ing to force the new wives to believe, just like they do to soldiers in Basic Training. The Army wants you to believe that the military takes care of their "own" and they use the catch phrase "mission first, people always." This phrase was a contradiction of terms. In reality, it was "mission always, people never."

It was at the AFTB that I met and befriended Maggie. She was a young soldier's wife -- "dependent" was the term used at the time. She was new to the military life and I took her under my wing. The installation was an alien and, often, cruel world, and I sensed that she needed guidance and protection. Maggie and I developed a close, mother-daughter kind of relationship.

At the American Red Cross, the Officers' wives reigned su-preme. Apparently, however, at some point they slipped up and let "one of those" slide in when I volunteered. The board position I had at the ARC threw me in with top commanders' wives and other influential people. It was an eye opening experience. During my service as a board member for almost five years, I learned that rules and regulations could also be bent and broken among the wives. Using organization funds for expensive farewell gifts was against the regulations, but it was understood that this rule could be bent in order to puff up the feathers of the big shots -- or the wanna be big shots.

At the other end of the spectrum, enlisted wives normally vo-lunteered for the Army Community Services (ACS) where they dealt with families in real distress. If a family member needed an emer-gency loan, because the military had failed to pay the soldier due to a computer foul up, the ACS is where they went for help. If a soldier found that military pay didn't stretch far enough to include groce-ries -- because the only available off post housing was more than his paycheck would allow -- the ACS is where he went. Officers' wives rarely dealt with these more mundane difficulties. They were better suited for rubbing elbows with the hierarchy than attending to the earthly needs of those who served under their husbands' commands. Besides, the ACS process was a degrading experience -- the paperwork, the way people stared at you, and the report that had to go back to the command. It was hard enough on these young soldiers and their families, who served their country for so little pay. Being forced into having to ask for assistance and knowing everyone would hear about it was a blow that most soldiers found embarrassing. It was common knowledge that a lot of lower enlisted soldiers and their families were on food stamps and received Medicaid. What most people didn't know about, however, was that it was not always the enlisted soldiers who asked for help. I helped a Captain and his family, who were struggling. He was mortified about asking for help, because of his rank, but he had no other choice. His family was hungry.

Living accommodations on the post were not a perfect situation either. Housing was not always provided for the soldiers and their family members. However, Maggie was one of the fortunate ones -- or was she? Her two-bedroom duplex was better than a slum apartment, but not by much. There was a three-inch gap between the baseboard and wall that ran the entire length and width of the living room. This made a perfect entrance for snakes and brown recluse spiders, of which both could be found in the dwelling on any given day. Then, there are the rules and regulations designed to keep the tribe members in line, while living on the installation. For example, the Post Engineers (DPW) came around and wrote citations if the grass was a half an inch too high or if one had more than the permitted three animals living in the duplex. As a cat lover, this was too restrictive for me. Tim and I decided to live off post.

The military has an agency called Post Housing. This agency is supposed to ensure that the off-post soldiers were treated fairly and that their quarters were up to the military's (obviously low) standards. Unfortunately, we learned that Post Housing did not take its responsibility too seriously. The military kept a list of all the local unfair businesses. This was called the black list. When our black-listed landlord failed to repair the large, gaping holes in the garage doors that left us vulnerable to theft, we called Post Housing to complain. An inspector was sent out, agreed that the holes should be patched up, and filled out a report. Then, we waited. No matter how many times we called Post Housing to insist that the inspector deal with the landlord as promised, nothing more was ever accomplished. When the air-conditioning went out in 112-degree weather, nothing was done to remedy this situation either. Since every incident report made its way to the soldier's command, we learned to pick our battles carefully to avoid being labeled as troublemakers. Eventually, we simply moved instead of forcing the issue.

There were serious responsibilities that came with being the Family Support Group leader. When I took over the group, I responded to each task seriously, especially when reporting on something being amiss in a family in the unit. One day, a soldier's wife asked me to come to her home. I agreed and met her that afternoon. She said that she had something to tell me. I stopped her before we went any further. I need to know whether I was there in my AFTB or FSG capacity or whether I was just there as a fellow military wife. I explained that with each option came a different obligation. As the AFTB instructor, I could provide resources or explain which avenue to take, but I had no authority to report anything to command. If I was there as the FSG leader, I had a duty to report whatever I learned to the command. And, as just another military wife, all I could offer her was a supportive ear. The woman thought about her options for a few minutes and then asked me to be there in my FSG role.

She suspected her husband of sexually abusing her four year-old daughter from a previous marriage. She wasn't sure what to do about the situation since he was a senior NCO (Non Commissioned Officer), and he had convinced her that a soldier's laundry stayed in his own basement. I began to jot down notes and ended up taking three pages of information. The man accused was my husband's team leader. So, I knew that this would prove to be a sticky situation.

I called my minister that evening and discussed my dilemma in confidence. If I reported this to the civilian authorities, it would become public knowledge and the military would lose face. If I reported this to the military command, as I had been instructed to do through training, the military would still look bad. There was never any question in my mind that the situation had to be reported, but I had hoped there might be an easier solution to the problem. The minister, who was also an active duty military officer, advised me to go through the chain of command, starting with the OIC (Officer in Charge) of the unit.

The OIC was a Major and had always appeared to be a fair and impartial man. He and I were on first name basis and worked closely on many occasions. I was not thrilled to be bringing him this information, but knew what I had to do. I wouldn't ask him to handle the situation. I knew in my heart that I must see this through myself to the end.

When I went to speak to the Major, he invited me into his dingy, dull office. There was barely room for his desk, swivel chair, and the two wooden chairs that were placed six inches in front of his desk. The quarters were cramped, to say the least. I was directed to take the seat furthest from the door. As was his habit, the Major asked a retired Command Sergeant Major to chaperone the conversation. It was a general rule of thumb not to be alone with another soldier's wife at any time for any reason. I had an appointment with Social Services on post in a couple of hours so I got right to the point of my visit.

"Sir, something has come to my attention as the FSG leader and it involves one of your soldiers," I blurted out.

"Who is the soldier?" the Major asked, wrinkling his brow.

I gave him the soldier's name and explained the situation, referring to my notes for accuracy. The Major leaned back in his chair, clasped his hands together and the room suddenly became deathly quiet. It seemed that this turn of events had taken him by complete surprise.

The retired CSM was next to speak. "Are you sure the wife is telling you the truth about this?" he asked.

It sounded like he was implying that the soldier's wife might have cause to take revenge in this vicious way for something the command may already be aware of. I told him that I could not be sure about the accuracy of her story, but since she had reported it to me, I took it seriously, as should they. At this time, I made the two men aware of my intentions.

This news brought the Major to his feet. He leaned over the desk and glared at me. He was livid. I had never witnessed such an outburst from any officer and certainly never from the Major.

"Do you realize what you are doing?" he bellowed. "You are about to ruin a soldier's career!"

Offended by his demeanor, I stood up to leave, but the body filling the chair next to me blocked my way. It was clear that they were not finished with trying to sway me from taking this information outside of the room. I felt as if the walls were closing in.

Then, the officers took turns -- one yelling and the other firmly commanding that I drop this and let them handle the situation. This went on for almost two hours until they were finally worn down and satisfied that I would not change my course. I left that office even more determined to get this incident behind me. I was doing what was right and believed that I had nothing to fear by taking responsibility for my leadership position.

After word made it through the chain of command, Tim was called on the carpet in front of his direct superior. This man told Tim that I was not doing the right thing and would probably ruin the soldier's career. He went one step too far. He instructed my husband to "take charge of his wife and keep her under control." He might as well have said that I was responsible for this soldier allegedly abusing his stepdaughter. He further implied that any soldier should be able to control of his wife no matter what the situation. It was as if wives were a piece of equipment, and the soldier could force the equipment to operate in the way the military wanted it to work --invisibly and quietly. I saw this woman and her husband many times at the Social Service office waiting for their caseworker, but I never heard if the soldier was found guilty or innocent. It was to stay forever hushed up.

On many occasions after this incident, the same Major and Tim's direct supervisor would call me to request favors. I was asked to teach an emergency class or arrange an event for the unit. I always obliged. I had my hopes that they learned something as valuable as I did from that experience. I learned that no matter what, doing the right thing gives you strength and character.

While the Major had taken command of another unit across the post and I had not seen him for months, the Major and I would cross paths again. Maggie's husband was under the Major's command now, and it looked like John was having an affair with a female soldier in another unit. If John's actions were proven, it would be grounds for severe punishment by the military.

John moved from their duplex into the barracks and Maggie asked for my assistance in uncovering the truth. I indulged her, but I never suspected John as the type of guy who would cheat on Maggie. He didn't fit the profile of a dishonorable soldier.

Maggie and I scheduled surveillance time together and kept notes on the process. We visited parking lots to locate the female's car, so we would have a picture of it for the records since it was seen driving past Maggie's duplex on a nightly basis. We made inquiries of other members of her unit and found that she had emotional problems. When Maggie reported to John's command about her suspicions, they turned a deaf ear. She had no actual proof to present, and they would not flag a soldier on unsubstantiated charges. Maggie wanted to find that proof. She saw it as her only way to end the affair and tether her husband back into the relationship he had strayed from. She believed that was the best solution for both of them.

One afternoon, Maggie found letters and poems that John and his female friend had exchanged. She found her proof. Maggie called the command and spoke to the duty desk soldier.

"Is the Commander in?" Maggie asked.

"Negative," the desk soldier responded in typical military parlance.

"Would you please take a message for him?" she asked.

"Yes, Ma'am," the soldier said.

"He knows what this is about," Maggie explained. "I want a federal investigation started and I have proof now."

After her phone call with the command, Maggie felt relieved. Now something could be done to right this wrong situation. This would happen eventually, but not before the Central Intelligence Division (CID) got involved in the case. This is an agency I would compare to the FBI in civilian life.

A few days after Maggie's message to the Commander, my doorbell rang. I was busily preparing for a twelve hour teaching marathon. I looked haggard and was not up to having any company. I peered out the peephole and saw two Jehovah's witnesses. The gentleman was dressed in a dark trench coat and black shoes. His hair was longer than the usual military cut, but every strand was firmly in place. The female was wearing Salvation Army type shoes. Her straight, black skirt hit well below her knees and her gray jacket fell below her hips. Her glasses were non-military, but just as unattractive and her hair was short and slightly disheveled. After one look, I decided not to answer the door. But the couple at the front door persistently rang the bell, until out of pure annoyance, I opened the door.

"I am not interested," I told them as politely as possible and started to close the door.

"Ma'am, we are from the CID," the agent spoke as he flashed his identification. "We want to come in."

I opened the door wider while I took this all in. I thought to myself, "Now, what the hell could I have done that would warrant the CID to be at my front door?"

The agents sat tentatively on the sofa. The female noticed my artwork and commented briefly. The man was all business and immediately explained the reason for their visit.

"Ma'am, we have a report that you and a Maggie Smith called the Commander, posing as Federal Agents," he stated.

It felt like an eternity before I was able to absorb his statement, and even longer to formulate a reply.

"What the hell are you talking about?" I asked. I was stunned.

"Ma'am, we received the information from a reliable source. You made a telephone call stating that you were a Federal Agent," he replied matter-of-factly.

"Your reliable source is evidently not as reliable as you believe it is," I retorted. Knowing this was an absurd accusation, I was angry. How dare they accuse me of such an action!

"We will be back later to arrest you, Ma'am," he threatened, making his way towards the front door.

"Well, you just do that!" I said. "When you come back, you had better have better proof, because this is nonsense."

I called Maggie immediately. I knew they would be talking to her next, if they hadn't already.

"Mags, there are two CID agents on their way to your house," I spilled out. "They were just here and accusing ME of making a call posing as a Federal Agent!"

John and Maggie were waiting for them. The male agent commented that he was sure I would call her about their visit. He was right. This was the most idiotic situation of all the situations I had seen the military cook up. That evening, no one came to arrest me.

The next morning, I called JAG (Judge Advocate General). I explained what had happened and asked for their assistance in clearing up this matter. I was told that it would be six weeks before a standard investigation could be completed, and that I would be notified of the outcome at that time. I couldn't wait six weeks when the only outcome would be that the CID had made a grave mistake. My next stop would be the office of the CID Commander. I picked up Maggie and off we went.

At the CID intake window, I gave my name and asked to see whoever was in charge. It was obvious that they were not expecting us. A brief call and a sharp buzzer, we were through the locked glass doors and inside the secretive world of the CID. I was too filled with anger to be impressed.

A short, thin black woman met us at the doors. As she directed us to follow her to an office, she explained that she was the person in charge. We walked down hallways, past other agents obviously working cases, and through another set of double doors. As we started down the last dimly lit hallway, I noticed prison cells along one wall.

"Hey, Maggie, better pick one out before all the good ones are taken," I whispered jokingly.

Maggie was nervous and she tugged on my shirt from behind. My humor was lost on her, as I heard her sob quietly. I gave her a courageous smile and quieted her tears.

Evidently, the office was not one that was used for work. It was a spacious room with a desk and a few chairs scattered about, and it had that chemical smell of newly installed carpeting. Maggie and I took seats. The woman in charge took a seat behind the desk and propped her feet up on it.

She tilted back in her chair and said, " I know why you're here."

"I don't know where these charges came from," I said, "But I want to get this cleared up immediately."

The woman didn't speak, so I continued. "I've already spoken to JAG, but I think waiting six weeks to find out that these are false allegations is way too long."

To my surprise, she nodded in agreement. "The charges were dropped yesterday," she stated in a way that implied we should have already known that piece of information. "The investigators knew from your responses to their visit that there was a misunderstanding somewhere and they learned what really took place."

"Is anyone going to tell us what actually took place?" I asked.

"The soldier on the desk took down the message that Maggie called in," she began, eyeing me carefully. "It seems that because Maggie wanted a Federal investigation, he wrote down that you were Federal Investigators," she chuckled. "The soldier was questioned and admitted that he noted the wrong information," she finished her explanation by standing up.

"Do you mean to tell me that if that soldier had not admitted to his mistake, this investigation would have continued?" I asked.

"Yes, I'm afraid so," she replied, ushering us back the way we came in. "But, I am sure we would have gotten to the bottom of it eventually."

Once we were outside in the parking lot breathing fresh air again, Maggie admitted that she had been so frightened that she had almost wet herself. Isn't life grand?

CHAPTER II

Military Healthcare and Antics

In May of 1997 just before our first anniversary, I developed the worst case of the flu that I had ever experienced. I was so ill that I had to call into work for the day off, something I never did.

"You looked fine yesterday," said the doctor, who ran the lab I worked for as an office manager. "If you aren't dying, I strongly suggest you report for work," he stated.

His words only frightened me, because I felt like I was dying. Instead of going to work, I made a same-day appointment to see my Primary Care Physician (PCP).

"Last Four?" the desk clerk asked abruptly. "Last Name?" she continued in the same gruff manner.

Anyone who has ever been around the military knows the routine. We are not considered people -- just numbers and a last name.

The desk clerk directed me to an uncomfortable seat to wait for the next attendant.

In the intake room, the blood pressure cuff never fit properly and the attendant's standard questions seemed absurd. The requested information was already written in bold black ink on the front of my medical records. On a previous visit, I had asked why this inquest was necessary considering that he already had the answers in front of him. He responded that it was to ensure that I was really who I said I was. I pointed out that my name was also printed in bold black ink and the front desk clerk had already matched my mug with the photo on my military dependent identification card. The rolling eyes and pursed lips of the attendant told me that any further conversation about the long-standing procedure would be considered grounds for rebuff. I knew I would never get a logical or intelligent answer. This was how it was always done. End of discussion.

My PCP, Dr. Andrews was a teddy bear of a man. He was British, with a gentle manner, and believed in total patient care. Every visit began with a conversation about how my job was going, how my husband was doing and if there was anything new in our lives. This gave him a clear picture of the whole person sitting in front of him.

"What brings you in today, Sue?" he asked.

"The flu," I responded. "And I need a referral to the Dermatology Clinic for this rash."

Dr. Andrews flipped through my medical records, reviewed the last visit notes, and asked me about my symptoms. At first, the visit seemed like a routine one. I reported a fever, body aches, and fatigue. Dr. Andrews took notes and asked to see my rash. There were three bull's eye circles on my upper left arm, one fairly large. He immediately excused himself and returned just as promptly with two other clinic physicians. Clearly, this was not a routine visit any more. I couldn't imagine what could be so interesting about my rash.

The thick medical journal was flopped opened and the three physicians huddled around it. Their hushed but eager enthusiasm reminded me of teenage boys looking at a centerfold from a girlie magazine in an old 50's movie. One doctor would look closely at the book and then carefully examine my rash. Then, the next would repeat this process until all three appeared to be satisfied.

"No doubt about it," they muttered, bobbing their heads like hula-dolls in the back of a car window. "It's Lyme Disease."

The medical journal recommended Doxycycline and Motrin be administered. I never did get the referral for the Dermatology Clinic.

"I want to run a couple of lab tests to rule out other possibilities," said Dr. Andrews. "The results should be back in a week or so."

When the doctor called me with the lab results, I learned that I didn't have Multiple Sclerosis, Rheumatoid Arthritis, Diabetes, and that my thyroid looked okay. But, there was an indication that I was borderline Lupus. Dr. Andrews did not seemed concerned. He asked that I stop in for a Lyme titer in a week or two.

I had been on antibiotics for almost a month now and the Lyme titer came back negative. With hindsight, I now know that Lyme titers are almost always negative due to the effect of antibiotics. The doctor told me to come back, if I developed other symptoms or if I felt worse.

Over the next four years, I would compile a long list of symptoms, experience pneumonia yearly, and take many other medications in addition to the Doxycycline and Motrin.

Early in 1998, I noticed increased fatigue. It was so bad that I had to curtail many activities. I was even too tired most mornings to get out of bed. I traded in my hectic calendar for a lighter schedule.

There were a lot of changes being made on Ft. Sill. One of these changes was at our commissary. The rules were being bent to allow non-military inside the store now. For as long as anyone can remember, the commissary had always been off limits to civilians. But, sales were slumping. Promoting this as "good will" was a way to get around the regulation. Management turned their heads knowing that civilians were now shopping in the exclusive store.

Tim was taking over as Section Chief for another unit. He wasn't looking forward to this, but in the military there's no such thing as job choice. We found that if we were suffering something unpleasant, we always said, "this too shall pass". Eventually, it does pass, and we learn something from the experience. This time, the lesson would come with a price tag.

This was not an easy transition. We were not welcomed. In fact, I didn't meet anyone in the new unit for months. It wasn't until the former FSG leader called me and asked if I would be interested in helping out that I began to meet the new unit.

Tim was in charge of a few soldiers now. The job description did not sound difficult to me. This was supposed to be the last leg before retirement for us. As usual, we would make the best of it.

Tim was just getting settled into his position. The previous chief was walking him through the procedures and paperwork. It was soon time for the chief to leave for another assignment. The last detail to finalize the exchange was a signing over of the equipment.

The paperwork looked in order and the exchange was rushed. Training exercises and other military duties kept each soldier busy and away for weeks at a time. Tim signed without the requested inventory. The act was swift and sealed.

Tim was busy constantly. It was nothing for the unit to be training for two weeks out in the field, then back on post for a week or so, and then back out to the field. The next ten months flew by and it was time to make another exchange of chiefs.

This time training and unit demands for the soldiers were more lax, and there would be a full inventory. Tim learned that there was equipment missing. In fact, he heard that the equipment had been missing when the last chief was in charge. But, Tim had signed for everything when he took over as chief, including the missing items.

Some tools and part of a shelter (tent) were the missing items. The total came to $1,200. Tim paid the bill out of his own pocket and the exchange was made. We learned never to trust anyone, especially when pressed for time.

This same unit needed FRG leadership. I volunteered to take it for a short time -- just long enough to set the established rules and get a few meetings under our belts. When the BC (Battery Commander) is weak, as he was in this unit, the job of a good FRG leader was a tough mission. The entire program had to be typed, including what the BC was supposed to say. The other speakers had to be scheduled, and refreshments needed to be arranged. I happened to be fond of the BC and his wife. He confided in me one day that he never wanted a command. I understood why he was a weak leader -- the desire was not there.

The outgoing FRG leader had the journals that held all the accounting for every cent earned for the group. I was asked to sign for the books. Once I took a look at them, I decided not to sign anything until an audit was performed. Something wasn't right.

While a call for an audit was unheard of, it was well within my rights. I caught a rash of nasty emails from the First Sergeant and his wife, and I was shunned by the BC, who was the military leader of the FRG. Word spread quickly and the unit became divided.

The internal audit was to be conducted by a Major in the unit. He was one of the nicest men I knew and his wife and I were close friends. This would have no bearing on the audit, but at least I was sure that it would be a fair one.

The audit took over a week and the results confirmed my suspicions. There was money missing and the BC was responsible for it. I knew that a $200 cash amount that I had personally given him was not entered into the journal, triggering my suspicions in the first place.

The BC was ordered to repay the missing funds and I was fired from the volunteer position -- not necessarily the fair outcome I had anticipated.

Shortly before our second anniversary, on Labor Day weekend on 1998, all of my flu symptoms returned. This time, they were worse. Two days would pass before I was coherent enough to learn that my fever had spiked to 106 degrees. My feverish chills had required seven quilts on top of an electric blanket. In my delusional state, I ranted about a cat being on the backyard fence. My husband had found me in this condition when he came home from duty that evening. He immediately called my friend, Julie, who was a nurse. Experience told Tim that a trip to the military hospital would entail more than a six-hour wait before I could even see a physician. Julie was able to bring my fever down and Tim sat by my side until I came around. When I called Dr. Andrews to report the incident, he had me come in right away -- no appointment needed. I told the doctor that all three bull's eye rashes had reappeared that morning and I had experienced the flu symptoms again. That was all I remembered. Another Lyme titer was done. Again, it came back negative. Dr. Andrews could only follow the procedures in place for testing. The Center for Disease Control's (CDC) test criteria was a positive titer first, and then, and only then, a Western blot would be performed. In the military, one does not question procedures or protocols -- even if they are absurd.

Later, I learned that in the same year I had been infected, the Navy had been monitoring ticks at various installations. Their findings were that 16 military and a total of 12,801 cases of Lyme Disease were reported to the CDC. My doctor knew I had Lyme Disease in 1997. Now, I wondered if it had ever been reported to the CDC.

Being stationed in Oklahoma was not an easy tour. The weather was unbearably hot and the wind never stopped. It was not uncommon to see blue Wal-Mart bags intertwined in the rows of fencing, along with discarded newspapers and burger wrappers. The grass ranged from a sad green to a deadened brown year round. During the summer months, the air-conditioning in my truck broke. I began to notice increased wooziness, headaches, joint pain, and moodiness. My days were pure torture now. When I spoke with Dr. Andrews about these agonizing symptoms, he chalked it up to stress and long hours at work. I "worked" more rest into my schedule and increased my medications. I was convinced that this disease just needed time to run it its course and I would simply have to be patient.

Then, I suffered my first of many cases of pneumonia. It started innocently enough. I felt more tired, but I always suffered fatigue. I noticed that I was having a little trouble breathing and my energy was more strained than usual. I tried to rest more, but the symptoms were not easing up. Another doctor's visit was in order.

Dr. Andrews was concerned. He ordered an X-ray and pointed out that there was fluid in my lungs. He prescribed Biaxin for ten days and sent me home. Within two weeks, I found myself in the emergency room of the military hospital. The wait would be almost six hours after another X-ray and I never even saw a doctor. The nurse informed me that the doctor on call reviewed my x-ray and instructed me to call my PCP Monday morning for an appointment. This was Friday night! But, I complied and Tim drove me home.

Julie stopped by after her shift at the civilian hospital. She wanted to chat, but I was just not up to it. I could barely catch my breath and things were spinning. Julie listened to my chest, took my temperature, and called an ambulance. This time, the doctor would not be able to put me off.

The ambulance drivers got lost, and had me direct them from our subdivision to the hospital. Tim and Julie made it to the emergency room before the ambulance. The wait to see a doctor was longer than what I would expect in the emergency exam room, but he finally came in.

"Aren't you the same woman that was here earlier?" the doctor asked gruffly.

"Are you the same doctor that sent me home without seeing me when I was here earlier?" I retorted.

Round one. Ding!

There were labs to be done and I learned that the doctor wanted yet another X-ray. This seemed like a waste of time, as he had just done one earlier that day. I was sure that nothing much could have changed in that short a time. I refused to have it done. I volunteered at this hospital to save them money. I would not allow someone to waste funds on my account. Blood was drawn and I was left alone.

Round two was about to begin.

"I'm having blood gases drawn," the doctor dictated.

I knew that blood gases were not necessary for pneumonia and that the procedure was a painful one. This was just as unwarranted as a second X-ray. "You are not drawing blood gasses," I told him firmly.

"You are the patient and I am the doctor," he barked, storming out of the bay.

"Get me another doctor," I requested, looking at the nurse.

It just so happened that two doctors that I knew very well were in the emergency room on other business. One of these men, Dr. Thompson, was the head of all the clinics at the hospital. I must have been holding my mouth right, as my grandmother used to say. This was my lucky day.

Overhearing the ruckus, Dr. Thompson came to my bedside and asked what was going on. I explained what had transpired, he agreed with my call, and suggested that I file a report against the ER doctor. He would back me up.

Dr. Thompson admitted me to the hospital where I stayed for three days of intensive IV and breathing treatments. I was very grateful to finally be treated. When I was released, I felt better than I had in months. I didn't know what lay ahead on my journey through the maze of Lyme Disease, but I was in for the ride, literally, for my life.

The first significant episode of disorientation commonly associated with Lyme disease occurred one evening after Tim and I had gone out to dinner. I slid behind the driver's seat and headed home. Suddenly, on the four-lane highway I had traveled daily, I was forced to stop. This was not merely a moment of forgetfulness. I was completely lost. Nothing looked remotely familiar and I was terrified. Tim was gentle and patient. He spoke softly and calmly giving me directions home, as if he were speaking to a child.

After this scare, I began trying to explain my symptoms to anyone who would listen. I had always found that whenever I mentioned an affliction to another person, they either have had the same illness or know of someone suffering from it. But no matter whom I spoke with, no one shared my symptoms. I suddenly felt very alone and for the first time in my life, I began to question my own state of mental health. I was sure I just needed a distraction.

My hospital stay left me well enough physically to take on a happy project to cheer me up. Every year, the civilian community had decorated the median in the downtown area and it became a winter wonderland with carriage rides, a Santa shack, animated displays, lights of every color, and larger than life angels that were lit up on tall poles to watch over the visitors. I was hired as the project manager. It was not much money, but it would brighten my world.

The project started off badly. I had been told that the contacts would be made to ensure that I had volunteers to assist me in this somewhat daunting task. This was clearly a misunderstanding, as there were no civilian volunteers. Luckily for me, I was well connected. One phone call to the post and soldiers were there the next morning and every weekend thereafter.

There was a woman who was hired to be my assistant, but I was disappointed in the board's choice. This woman cared more about making eyes at the volunteer soldiers than she did about working. She would show up late or not at all. She collected her paychecks, but she definitely did not earn the money. When it would come time to take the decorations down, she never bothered to return to finish the job.

After that experience, I no longer desired to volunteer my time to the community during the most sacred time of the year. Their winter wonderland became a winter Wasteland. That was the last year I saw the Christmas display.

Tim was gone more than usual. His Army career kept him

away six to eight weeks at a time, teaching the AFATADS system to soldiers in other states. I noticed that I began to be increasingly more irritated at him. With my neurological symptoms of Lyme Disease on the increase, my world was tilting off its axis and I could do nothing to stop it. I felt like I was losing my mind and there was no relief in sight.

When our soldiers are away it is the military wives' tradition to rearrange the furniture. This is as an important tradition as any Hail and Farewell held in honor of incoming and outgoing soldiers. I noticed that more energy was necessary for me to move the sofa. It took longer for me to rearrange things. And I had difficulty working out a plan for the layout. It was becoming obvious that I was losing my strength, stamina, and thought process. I was being slowly robbed of my well being, and I became angrier and more stressed by the minute.

During this time, Tim had a mini-stroke on the running track during a physical fitness test. He was rushed to the military hospital, which released him at once, saying they could find nothing wrong with him. I asked my employer, a cardiologist, to have a look at him, since his symptoms were not uncommon to the stroke patients we saw in the office. After an exam, my boss diagnosed him as having had a mini-stroke. This was not good news. He was immediately flagged and within weeks, removed from the promotion list. He was devastated and this sent him into a depression that would last for over two years. Now we were BOTH sick!

I was only forty-four, but I knew how someone one hundred and forty-four felt might feel. My vision was getting blurry, my back hurt with every twist or turn, and my hands were numb and tingly. My body creaked and cracked; it sounded like my bones would break at any given moment. My lungs felt heavy and I had developed a cough. I was almost afraid to call Dr. Andrews. I was sure he would refer me for a psychological exam instead of the annual visit. When the brain fog lifted from time to time, I would question my own sanity. How could anyone have all these symptoms and not be crazy?

It would turn out that I was not insane. However, after filling out the paperwork to enroll in the Exceptional Member Family Program (EFMP), that the military insists be completed for each dependent, I learned that maybe I was, at the least, an oddity. The

EFMP is supposed to assure that when a soldier is under consideration for a change in duty stations, the enrolled family member is taken into account. This doesn't guarantee that the soldier won't be sent to a post that can accommodate the family member, but we were told that a family member's medical needs would be taken into account when making the final decision. As this story unfolded, I found that no consideration was given pertaining to my medical needs.

In September of 2000, Tim came down on orders. Okay, it wasn't Germany or Italy, but South Korea would be an interesting duty station. But not for me, as it turned out. This was an unaccompanied, year-long tour. My symptoms were listed on the EFMP paperwork and PERSCOM (the command that regulates military personnel) knew that Tim was the only help I had in the world. Yet, the military was sending him thousands of miles away and leaving me to fend for myself with Lyme Disease. Once a soldier leaves the post, the remaining family members are no longer visible in the eyes of the military. We are baggage that they do not want around. We are no longer attached to a unit or any Family Support Group. We are solely our spouse's responsibility, but our spouse is no longer there!

Have you ever seen a magician do rope tricks or pull a rabbit out of a black top hat? You may have seen some wonderful magicians in your time, but never any as good as what the military has. The military may not put on a show with rabbits and magic wands, but it's quite a show nonetheless.

There was a lower enlisted soldier named Ernie, who was always having problems in the military. He had entered the Army life with no less than eighteen misdemeanors -- when three was the military limit. After an argument with his wife, Ernie brought his own civilian weapon to the post, which is a federal offense. Ernie was always in debt and could never pay his bills. One would think that his actions and previous misdemeanors would have been enough to discharge him from the military. Instead, he came down on orders for South Korea! Someone in command had either missed these important facts or chose to ignore them. Ernie's orders left the command scrambling to get him clearance for this tour. The command was ready for this soldier to become someone else's problem and they would jump through any necessary hoops to get this soldier to South Korea. One day, out of the blue, Ernie had his clearance. The charges against him had not been dropped; they had simply vanished from his records. However, when Ernie came back from his tour in South Korea, looking forward to enrolling in a technical school, he was denied enrollment. His misdemeanors had suddenly reappeared on his records. These were some powerful magic tricks!

While I quietly questioned my own sanity from the neurological effects of Lyme Disease, I also began to question the sanity of the actions on the military post.

In the hours after 9/11, paranoia swept the battalions. Doors were chained shut, with the exception of the main and 'command entrance only' entrances. Guards were posted at each entrance (even though they were chained and locked). Barricades and barbed wire were set up with no parking within 50' of any building. Complete ID searches were conducted at the motor pool and battalion headquarters entrances. And roving guards carried empty rifles. The ammunition was considered too dangerous. Soldiers were not supposed to shoot anyone -- just display their weapons and hope they scare the enemy into surrendering. Or, maybe the bullets were too expensive since legacies would prove to be more important.

The Command Sergeant Major (CSM) at this unit believed that tablecloths were certainly more important than bullets. Leaving a legacy was a common dream among Command Sergeants Major. Every legacy had to become a living memorial of their command. However, the CSM at this post could only be classified as a waste of sperm. He was a biased, egotistical, self-centered, uncaring, and politically motivated racist. Everything that happened had to revolve around him and become his business. His job was actually the senior ranking, enlisted advisor to the commander. Instead, this CSM believed that he ran the command, enlisted or otherwise. His way, according to regulations or not, was the only way. And, he was out to leave his legacy at any cost.

These tablecloths were gaudy, too. They were the brightest red and trimmed in a fake, flashy gold fringe. And all to the tune of $3,000.00 of taxpayer money.

The CSM wasn't done yet. He had one more legacy he wanted to leave -- SIGNS! One sign was ten feet high by twelve feet wide. Very impressive compared to the other motor pool signs around post and totally against post regulations. The whole sign only cost taxpayers $1,300. It showed an undignified lack of respect for the backbone of the unit, which consists of the enlisted soldiers -- not the CSM.

But, no one complained. Not the soldiers, who were struggling to make ends meet. Not the families, who were on food stamps because the military doesn't pay well enough or had failed to pay due to a glitch in the system. Not even the FRG leader, who couldn't sell hot dogs to raise funds for a group event because it was against post policy to be so near a soda machine (owned and operated by AAFES (Army Air Force Exchange/Extortion Service.

Everything seemed to boil down to whomever held the pen that wrote the orders and the checks. Those who served as the backbone of the military didn't have money to spend on tablecloths and signs. The legacy that the enlisted soldiers can afford to leave is the knowledge of a job well done -- even though they rarely hear those words spoken aloud.

I began to wonder where the fine line of mental health in the military life could be drawn -- or if it could be drawn at all.

CHAPTER III

Life In Texas and South Korea

The Navy seemed to be under way with Lyme Disease from reports I read. Tim and I decided to do a little more of our own research before he left for South Korea. We found that in southern Texas, near a Navy installation, there was a doctor who was involved with a Lyme Disease clinical study. This was a start that we viewed as a way back to good health for me. It was a move that had to be made before Tim left for his last tour. Later, I would regret this decision.

Moving to Texas was no small feat. Tim and I had decided to move ourselves. This is known in the military as a DTY (pronounced DITY) move. It meant packing and loading the moving van; driving over 400 miles; locating a house, and unpacking. After hiring a pizza deliver man to help load; a delay along the trip due to a wheel catching on fire, and hiring a homeless veteran to help unload at the new house, we made it in only four days. Tim would have to go back to Ft. Sill for three months to finish paperwork to prepare him for the South Korean tour. This would be my chance to start visiting a new physician in hopes of getting well. And I would be able to gauge how my life would be without Tim.

Before Tim headed back to Oklahoma, we made an appointment with the new physician that I would be seeing for my healthcare. Tim and I agreed that Dr. Edger was more than competent. We interviewed him and went over my medical files as a team. He was genuinely concerned with my Lyme Disease and concurred that a clinical study would be in my best interest. The doctor assured Tim that I would be his in "good hands" while Tim was overseas.

I busied myself with unpacking while Tim finished his stint at Ft. Sill. The days grew warmer and slipped by quickly. Soon, it would be time for Tim to come to Texas for a 30-day leave (vacation in civilian life). It is quite common for soldiers to spend time with their families before going off to an unaccompanied duty station. We had plans to go back east to visit relatives for most of the leave time. It would be a bittersweet time in our lives.

I met Nickie not long after I was settled into the Texas house. She was an emotional woman, but I took pleasure in her company. One evening, Nickie and I were enjoying coffee and a pleasant conversation at my dining room table. Suddenly, I suffered excruciating pain, vomiting, and diarrhea. This episode lasted almost 15 minutes, but was not the first time I had experienced this. Nickie took me to the local hospital where the emergency room physician decided that it was simply constipation. She released me with a bottle of red liquid that I was to drink the following morning. I did not agree with her diagnoses, but I followed her instructions.

The next afternoon, I was suffering with the same symptoms as the previous day. This time, I called an internist who asked me to come in immediately. After listening to my complaints, he diagnosed me with gallstones. To be sure, he ordered a test for the following morning.

The test result confirmed that I had gallstones and I was admitted to the hospital for surgery just two days before Tim was to start his leave. The surgery went well and I was back home the same day.

Tim was grateful to leave Ft. Sill. He would finally get some rest and enjoy a month away from military life. He was only 19 months away from a permanent separation from the military, known as retirement. We planned a bond fire for his last day in the U.S. Army. We would roast hot dogs over the burning uniforms and discuss all the sights we wanted to see in Australia. But first, off to South Korea after the leave and the remaining seven months spent ACAPing (transition process back to civilian life). We were looking forward to this last leg of the military life.

Tim's first night back in Texas, we planned to celebrate with a dinner out and our trip being the only conversation. Our suitcases were packed and the truck was loaded with camping gear, with plans to be on the road early the following morning. Another set back in our plans came immediately after Tim paid the dinner check. I experienced the exact same symptoms that had only days ago indicated gallstones. This surely could not be since my gallbladder had been removed. Tim rushed me to the hospital and I was admitted. The diagnoses was a missed gallstone and we would just have to wait it out. TriCare (military health insurance), actually stated that they wanted me to go home and wait it out. However, being on a machine that administers medication made their wish mute. After almost a week, I was released, minus the gallstone.

The back-east visit was a mix of joy and sorrow. Relatives were happy to see us, but there were tears when we said our good-byes. It would be over a year before we saw them again.

It was time to put Tim on the plane to South Korea. This was not the first time I had seen my husband off at an airport. In the past, many of his eight-week missions had required him to fly. This time was different in that he would be gone for a year. It was a stressful situation for each of us and all too soon, he was gone.

Nickie kept me busy the first couple of months that Tim was in South Korea. We went for long drives and had even longer talks. She kept me motivated with sightseeing and her family outings. She had lost her husband to cancer a few years ago and had just started dating again. When she finally met someone, I saw less and less of her. I was happy for her, but I was alone again.

It was time to refill my medications. I had not heard anything about the Lyme Disease study but intended to discuss this with my doctor at the appointment.

Dr. Edger's office had relocated and the staff had been replaced with a crew of unprofessional women. The office was grimy and Dr. Edger was somehow different. It was almost as if he were possessed. His eyes darted around the room and he appeared jumpy. This did not seem to be the same doctor Tim and I had found so competent at the initial interview. I asked about refills and was denied most of the medications he had previously written prescriptions for just a month ago. I handed him Lyme Disease material that outlined my symptoms better than I could convey, but Dr. Edger refused to look at it. When I mentioned the Lyme Disease clinical study he had vowed to get me into, he got anxious.

"It's all in your head," he said, refusing to look at me directly. "The best thing I can do for you is give you a referral to a shrink."

I was confused. This was the same doctor that had assured my husband that I would be in good hands. Just a month ago, he had asked for information on Lyme Disease after he wrote my prescriptions. This same doctor confirmed, in writing to the military, that I had Lyme Disease and listed that I had difficulties with everyday activities. I did not understand what had happened to this man. I knew he had to be reported to my insurance company. If I could, I would make sure that no other military family member would have to see this doctor. TriCare took the report, but it fell on deaf ears. Nothing was ever done.

In June of 2002, South Korea was heating up. Tim had been assigned to Area I. With a P-3 profile (much like a physician's statement limiting physical activity) which prohibited him from running, marching, and jumping.   Assigning anyone with a P-3 profile to Area I was against military regulations. Area I was next to the DMZ and the North Korean border. The military never assigned anyone to this area for safety reasons. There had been a cease-fire agreement between the North and South Koreas for 50 years now. But should there be any break in that agreement, a profiled soldier would be left without full use of his body for a retreat. I suppose this is the reason Tim was assigned a low-profile job in Area I, handing out driver's licenses to young soldiers. He was initially sent to South Korea to train soldiers to use the AFTADS computer system. With the low-profile job, the military was insured that no one would find out about Tim's P-3 profile or thir error in assignments.

This was also an unaccompanied tour area. Yet, there were many families there and the military made every effort to accommodate these families. There were evacuation plans and soldiers were responsible for seeing that these families were accounted for. This was called Non-Combatant Evacuation Operation or NEO. This matter seemed to have a high priority. It looked as if regulations were bent or broken easily in South Korea, too. Out of sight, out of mind described how the Pentagon reacted to these transgressions.

A Command Sergeant Major's barbeque grill came up missing. The entire unit was yelled at and accused of stealing. They later learned that a South Korean National that worked on the installation had taken the grill. One evening, during that same time period, a young soldier was taking pleasure in the popular past time in South Korea, drinking. He ended up jumping from his third floor window trusting this would end his misery. The First Sergeant immediately called the entire barracks out for formation during a typhoon! He kept them at attention while he blamed each and every NCO for the soldier's fate. Tim was one of the NCOs and he didn't know the soldier who tried to end his life. The soldier ended up paralyzed and shipped back to the states. The matter was closed and never discussed again.

June 13, 2002, there was an accident involving two soldiers, an armored vehicle, and two teenage girls. An investigation into the misfortune was conducted by the military (Military Police Investigations and The Army Safety Center) and the KNP (Korean National Police). They proved this to be indeed an unfortunate accident. The road was narrow and visibility from the vehicle had been limited. These findings were reported, but protests by some 6,000 South Korean Nationals, mostly college students, began. There were incidents of Molotov cocktails being lobbed over the gates at selected posts, demonstrations outside military installations with a report of protesters breaking through the secured area at Camp Stanley, and even a military officer was stabbed. In response to the unrest, the military decided to change their findings from "innocent" to "vehicular homicide". If found guilty, the soldiers could be sentenced up to six years in prison and lose their careers. Tim asked me to contact the soldiers and offer their families support. Before I would hear from anyone, my name would be all over South Korea. Word spread quickly about anyone advocating for one of our own.

I wrote each soldier a letter. Within a week, I was contacted by one of the soldier's sister, Lynn. She explained that her brother, Mark was the TC (tank commander) implicated in the incident. She said that she was skeptical about my offer to help, but her brother had encouraged her to call me. After numerous conversations, Lynn and I became close. She was not familiar with the military life and wanted to learn all she could so she could help her little brother. Lynn and Mark agreed that since the military had already charged him with a crime after having found him innocent, Mark felt he could not trust the military to represent him. I offered Lynn the name of an attorney in Houston that could defend Mark. Guy Womack was a retired Marine and handled military cases in a no-nonsense fashion. He was the best in the country and available to travel to South Korea.

Lynn wanted the entire world to know that the U.S. Army in South Korea was unjustly accusing Mark. I agreed to get the story to the press for her. Soon, Lynn and I were being called for interviews. The Army Times printed a story after weeks of stalling. The Stars and Stripes ran a piece about the accident with quotes from us. Even a small Georgia newspaper carried the story. But the best coverage came from The Atlanta Constitution. The journalist was true to his word and omitted our locations. I was receiving death threats written in Korean through email and was concerned since I lived alone.

Sammy Parker, a Korean-American religious leader, emailed Lynn. It was my position to field all unsolicited contacts and I replied to Mr. Parker's letter. He was offering support and wanted Lynn to know that all South Koreans were not against Americans as they had been portrayed in the media. Mr. Parker would prove to be a facilitator with the South Korean newspapers and, I still keep in contact with this wonderful gentleman even today.

A fund raiser was planned for Mark's defense fund. I traveled by bus and joined Lynn and her family for the event. They were more than I had expected. Lynn and her husband were so down to earth and considerate. Their children were intelligent and gracious. And Lynn's mother was purely delightful. I was welcomed into their family immediately. A lovely, private bedroom was mine for the visit and delicious meals were prepared as a family unit. Lynn's mother and I would go for short walks through the neighborhood and talk about her son, Mark. She was worried about the outcome of the military trial. I would try to assure her that Mark would be just fine and everything was being done that could be done for him. Her health was not good and she could not imagine her son going to prison for an accident. She just didn't understand how this could happen to a soldier that had served his country for over 15 years. Lynn filled me in on Mark's background. He was divorced and had a son in Alabama. This never came out in any of the newspapers. Lynn thought it best to keep his past private life out of it. Towards the end of my stay, Lynn received a call from Mr. Parker. He wanted us to meet him. He had a check for the $1,000.00 to donate to Mark's defense fund and there were several South Korean journalists that wanted to interview us for a human interest article. After the call, Lynn and I hugged and jumped into Lynn's car.

The South Korean men were so polite. They took pictures of us and guaranteed their articles would illustrate the compassion we felt for the families that lost their children in the accident. They kept their promise. We all hugged, shook hands, and shed tears when it came time to part.

Guy Womack was in South Korea to speak with Mark. So far, I had yet to hear from the other soldier, Fernando. One evening, while Guy was still in South Korea, a call came from JAG (Judge Advocate General-the military legal system). It was a Major, a military lawyer, who had just come on board to represent Fernando. This gentleman explained that he had spoken to his client and was trying to persuade him to seek civilian council. The Major was calling to ask if I would help his client as I had Mark to find legal representation if Fernando could be convinced. This Major disclosed that he was unfamiliar with the case and was given very little time to prepare a defense. I told him that I would certainly consider the request, but would need more information about Fernando in order to complete the task. He assured me that details would be forthcoming should his client decide to accept his advice.

Clearly irritated, Tim called to tell me that the military was bending over backwards and totally ignoring regulations, to collect money for the girls' families. There were containers set up at the military shopping areas; mandatory collections during formations, and the offerings at the military churches were being given to the families, as well. Tim said this smacked of corruption. Due to this behavior, Tim decided to stay away from church services. A monument to be placed at the accident site was being planned by the military in honor of the girls, too. And rumors were that the U.S. Government had already made a large payment ($25,000.00 to each family) for the accident. In light of how the military was treating this situation, we were appalled. The same day, Lynn received a check for $100.00 from a retired Command Sergeant Major working in South Korea for the defense fund. I contacted this gentleman to thank him. We have kept in contact to this day. In 2003, his Christmas card again suggested we "hang tough" as he knew the current situation that we were facing.

Mark was confined to the barracks. There were posters displaying his picture and demands for the military to turn him over to the South Korean courts. Mark's life was in danger if he left the safety of his room. He was suffering depression, anxiety and had been having nightmares. Mark relayed that he would rather be working to take his mind off the accident and all that had transpired since.

During the protests, a young soldier was kidnapped. John was fresh out of AIT (Advanced Individual Training). This was his first assignment and a rude introduction to the seedy side of military life in South Korea. John was with two other young Privates on a public train in Seoul. All of a sudden, almost two hundred South Korean protesters confronted the soldiers and shoved leaflets in their faces. What happened next would take strength and composure on John's part.

He was taken to the college stadium and forced to watch a demonstration involving over 6,000 college students protesting the military's refusal to turn the "murderers" over to the South Korean justice system. Then, he was shoved to his knees and compelled to say that he agreed with these demonstrators and that the military should not be in South Korea. John's mother tells me that according to John, a handgun was placed at John's the back of his head during this videotaped situation. John was then physically forced to accompany the protesters to a local hospital to apologize for injuring a South Korean National. It later was learned that this man was faking his injuries.

John was then arrested by the NKP and taken to join the other two soldiers waiting to be interviewed and charged. They were released back to the military and waited for a court appearance. The South Korean justice system failed to follow through in the allotted time and the charges were dropped.

After the dust settled, John brought his new wife over to join him and extended his South Korean tour to the maximum limit. I still receive emails from John's mother and last I heard, the kids were homesick, but doing okay.

Guy kept us informed of his progress with Mark's case. He had also decided to assist the Major with Fernando's indictment, sharing anything that developed. During Guy's pre-trial discovery, he found that the military was withholding information that was pivotal in clearing the soldiers in the initial investigation. Guy demanded the evidence and a physical reenactment of the accident. It was also uncovered that there was a legitimate reason that this accident occurred, but it had nothing to do with the Mark or Fernando. The Captain who was in charge of Mark's unit had not followed regulations in preparing his troops for this convoy. There was also another convoy coming from the opposite direction, which made the road even more treacherous. Preparation would have made the schedule known and two convoys on the same road would have been avoided. The lack of preparation and the narrowness of the road (which should have been also revealed in the preparation process) made it unsafe. The Captain was present in the convoy and ultimately responsible for the accident. But it would be months before this man's name would come out. He was an officer and it appeared that two enlisted soldiers' hides equaled one officer's. The military already had their sacrificial lambs.

The soldiers were acquitted and immediately flown back the United States. Comments from soldiers stationed in South Korea said that Guy was a real bulldog. He came in, took charge, and won the case. His presence was intimidating, I was told. There were rumors that the Captain would be charged with failure to follow regulations resulting in a fatal accident. Last I heard, he was transferred and enjoying life.

This should have been viewed as a good deed. In causal conversation, Guy told me that I may expect some problems over getting involved. I took this as his reference to the nasty emails from unknown persons. However, the military does not take kindly to anyone that interferes with their affairs, whether they are right or wrong. We would soon feel the military's wrath.

CHAPTER IV

Bound By Military Red Tape

The first attempt at gaining a compassionate reassignment came in early September of 2002, while Tim was in South Korea. The paperwork included statements from the South Korean command's chaplain, my husband, my friend Nickie, and myself. We attested to facts in the case with regards to my illness. By the first part of October, the first of five rejections for this request was received. The U.S. Army declared Lyme Disease a chronic disease and not worthy of a compassionate reassignment. My husband was crushed while I became frightened.

Tim had been loyal to the Army for twenty years. He had worked while suffering with the flu; went to combat when he was, as most soldiers, scared; and held his behavior to a personal high standards because he was a soldier. Even after he had been taken off the promotion list illegally in 1998, forced to take jobs that he was not trained to do, he still held respect for the military. He had taken an oath to protect and defend. How was he supposed to protect and defend his own wife when he was handing out driver licenses in Area I of South Korea? For the very first time, he was disappointed with the U.S. Army and disgusted with the lack of compassion shown by PERSCOM. It would not be long before he became disgusted with the entire government.

On the other hand, I was left alone to deal with my debilitating disease and make the best of it. I felt as if I were being treated worse than any captured terrorist. At least they were receiving medical care and had soldiers looking out for their welfare. My soldier was thousands of miles away in an area he was not supposed to be and could look out for no one except soldiers that could not pass driving tests. Constant fear for his welfare and mine kept my stress level high. I came to learn that stress is one of the keys that unlock the fury of Lyme Disease inside our bodies. Stress was now my worst enemy and the military was behind it.

Tim knew I was weakening and the Lyme Disease was getting worse. I was now having severe torso pains that could not be explained, increased headaches, and fatigue that kept me bedridden most of the time. I could no longer drive and my only resource, Nickie was working in Mexico. My cognitive skills made it almost impossible for me to function. Tim must have known I was going to get "lost" in my own home while he was gone. He had taped our phone number and emergency phone numbers on each phone. This was a good plan, but some days, I could not remember who I should even call if the house was on fire. It was becoming chronic. Had I known that this disease could be maintained, as the military knew, it would never have been able to get to this stage. But I didn't know and had put my life in the hands of the "expert" military doctors. I would continue to trust the physicians, military and civilian. For a while anyway.

In mid October of 2002, Tim put in the paperwork for a mid-tour leave. He wanted to come back for twenty-four days and take me to get medical treatment. He stopped believing me when I assured him I could wait the four months for this tour to end. It would turn out that his plan would actually save my life.

On January 8th, Tim got off the airplane near midnight. He saw me and knew, he says, that I probably would not live long. He commented on my pastiness and how weak I appeared. Within five days, we would be sitting at the Branch Medical Clinic, Ingleside, Texas. This would be the start of a nightmare that would last well over one year.

The doctor was on her last day at this duty station. She flipped through some paperwork that had nothing to do with me and asked why I was there. I explained that I needed refills on my medications for Lyme Disease that I had had since 1997 and that I had pain that no one yet could diagnose.

"You should be cured of Lyme Disease," she said matter-of-factly. "You don't need anymore medications for that."

"I can't walk when I come off the medications," I almost cried. "I have tried and it always turns out the same."

"Where's that pain?" she asked, ignoring my explanation. "I can refer you to NAS (Naval Air Station) for the pain. I am only here for a few more hours and then I move on to another base."

She referred me for the next day, as promised. As I left the exam room, I said a prayer, "Dear God, please don't let her ever meet another person with Lyme Disease."

This woman looked as if she were fresh out of medical school. Didn't she know that there was no cure for Lyme Disease? What possessed her to even think there was a cure?

Tim was scheduled to see an internist while I was with a surgeon at the NAS. In South Korea, he was only able to be seen by a Physician's Assistant for his thyroid and depression complaints. There had been tests, but nothing had been done for his thyroid.

We each went to our clinic appointments and agreed to meet in the waiting area when we were finished.

My doctor was in his mid thirties and pleasant enough. He looked at my x-ray, saw the marked area and diagnosed it as a cyst. This all took over an hour. The first interruption was a woman wanting him to sign some papers outside of the exam room. Next two intrusions were phone calls. Then, it was a patient wanting to speak with him and he said he got "hung up" with another doctor. I am not sure he even knew who I was after all of this. By then, I was fed up with the experience. I didn't feel that enough time was spent on options or even discussing the tests he wanted. His last comment to me was that he was leaving for Iraq and would not be back for some time. However, another doctor would do the surgery. So, this appointment was useless.

My husband was not faring any better. The doctor refused to treat him saying that he wouldn't be here long enough. I could not believe what I was hearing. It was time for action.

I don't know if it was the frustration of my appointment or someone refusing to treat a soldier, or both, but the commander was summoned. We explained what had transpired with both appointments. When it looked as though nothing was going to be done about it (and nothing was ever done), I asked for a referral for each of us to an Army medical facility and my records. The battle was now on.

The medical records, I was told, belonged to the military and I was not allowed to have them. I brought them in and I told them that I was taking them with me. After an hour of arguing about the possession rights of my file, the commander offered to copy them. I was exhausted. Instead, I asked that they be returned to the Branch Medical Clinic. If they could get them back there. This was the last I ever saw anyone at a Navy medical facility. I was never so thankful to be out of the Navy's hands and back with our own branch of the military.

The referral was all red tape. I had to sign a statement from the U.S Navy that I refused treatment before I could go to an Army medical facility. Anything, so I could get out of the clutches of these people! When I received my medical file (which now never leaves my sight), the Navy had reworked it. Now, test results were missing, among other documents. When I called them about this, a sailor at the clinic said that they had straightened the records out because the Army had them "all messed up".

Tim was granted a six-day extension on his leave orders. Since Space-A (military transportation) was the reason he was six days late on getting him home, the South Korean command was generous enough to allow the extra time. Once again, we felt blessed.

My referral led me to Dr. Whitehead, Brooke Army Medical Center, San Antonio, Texas. It was January 30th and time was running out. Even with the extension, we had only a week to get me back on my feet. The doctor understood and scheduled a next day appointment with Dr. Goodman from the Gastro Intestinal Clinic right next door.

On the 31st, Dr. Goodman saw me, actually listened to my complaints, and scheduled tests as quickly as possible. The South Korean command was notified through the American Red Cross and a fourteen day additional extension was granted. This relieved some of the pressure of feeling like a race horse at the start gate.

From February 6-April 30, 2003, I had thirty-two tests, two surgeries, three hospital stays and a list of medications an arm long. There were a total of eleven doctors involved in trying to get me well within the allowed time restraints set down by the military. Dr. Goodman, in writing, gave me less than five years to live.

From January 8 through May 1, six physicians submitted requests for Tim to be reassigned, 27-days of extensions,53-days of attachments, 24-days original leave. During this time, four compassionate reassignment packets were submitted (by request of CCAD, the Pentagon, and IG) and refused three times (to date, we have never been informed of the outcome of the last packet). On March 16, AWOL status went into effect (even with a leave form that said Tim had 21 more days of legal days to be here). There were also two curtailments requested, one being denied and the other was lip service from the South Korean command. During this time, to get everything straightened out, there were many calls made; thirty-four to South Korea command, ten to PERSCOM, three to American Red Cross (they refused to send anything else), twenty-four to Ft. Sam Houston Personnel Office, ten to Senator Hutchinson's office and three to Senator Cornyn's office (who on May 6 was "livid" at the way we were being treated after seeing our documentation and the following day was not interested in helping us). Nothing smells worse than a cowardly fish. Lucky for me that I had been found to have serious lung problems after the last surgery (due to an overdose of medication during surgery). I was ordered to wear a CPAP and could not smell the odor of cover-up and cowards.

More calls, one hundred fifty-nine were made to CCAD, four congressmen (PA,OH,TX,NJ), Lyme Disease support organizations, the Inspector General's office, a lawyer, the military pay office (DFAS), Judge Advocate General, and the landlord. But the calls that brought the IG to their knees and angered them enough to call us (May 1)were the ones to The White House (three) and The Secretary of The Army (five).

On March 25, TriCare (the military insurance) sent a letter denying me a Lyme Literate Medical Physician (LLMD), but it took until July 15, 2003 before I would hear from the IG's office asking what I wanted with an LLMD. It was a token call as I have never again heard from them.

Between April 7 and April 24, I had a heart attack, was threatened and served with eviction papers, told that only South Korean command could clear pay up, and had to pawn my wedding rings in order to eat (we never recovered enough to be able to get them back). I received two "AWOL next of kin" letters. Received on April 17, the first was dated April 5 and postmarked April 9. The second one, arriving on April 18, was dated March 26 and post marked April 9. Talk about covering their asses! Guess they didn't expect me to notice this or actually keep the envelopes.

April 16th would turn out to be the worse day of my Lyme Disease struggle. On advice from The Pentagon and the local Judge Advocate General, we went to the IG's office at Ft. Sam Houston. We were literally held captive. Tim was not allowed to get my medications nor would anyone there help me, and we were not offered any reason for being held against our will. Instead, the staff watched me in agony gasping for each breath, crying hysterically with pain, and no one lifted a hand to help. No one even bothered to call an ambulance. I was left to suffer.

It turned out that the sly CSM had called the Military Police to take my husband in and have him shipped back to South Korea. If this CSM had asked us to go to the MP Station, we would have obliged. He didn't have to lie or sneak around. We were sure that whatever the Army instructed us to do was for our own welfare and this would all be cleared up. Luckily, the M.P. that came was one soldier that used his good common sense (he also used it to get out of the military a few weeks later). He called a local unit and arranged for my husband to be attached there until PERSCOM decided on the outcome of the last compassionate reassignment paperwork (still no word after a year).

May 2003 was a really hard month for us. We were dirt poor, being evicted, had no health insurance (which meant that I could not get any medical help at all), and now having to sell everything we owned just to get a roof over our heads and a few meals. I cried at having to part with the only keepsakes left to me by my grandparents. It was one thing to lose my wedding rings to the pawn shop because we could not afford to get them out, but to part with the only piece left of my grandparents that raised me was the most difficult pill to swallow. This pain attacked my heart, but was even deeper than any heart attack I could ever experience.

Tim's commander (retired) from Ft. Sill and his wife sent us a check for $50.00. They understood what kind of people we were and knew that if Tim had stayed to help me through an illness (and I allowed him to do it for me), then it was serious. We had always been, in the eight years they had known us, good military people and ones who followed the rules.

The last slaps in the face were being evicted like a couple of deadbeats and then, not having enough gas money to make a short trip to funerals of two relatives who died a day apart. We were reduced to feeling as though we were crust on the bottom of an old tossed out Army boot. Guess this is one way to say "thank you" to a soldier who has given over twenty years and a wife who supported the military in any way, shape or form.

We loaded up our vehicle with the few things we had left and headed out. We did not know exactly where we were going or what we would be challenged with next. But, we had no home, no insurance, no income, I was so sick, and we barely had enough money to get anywhere. Our families were so small and none of them in a position to help us with any of these difficulties. We were on our own and we took this as a trial of our survival skills.

I rationed my medications, not knowing when I would ever get anymore. We started eating one small meal a day and went dumpster-diving for things we needed. We passed "embarrassed" after the first day on the road when we split a meal in a tent and fought back tears because we were cold.

CHAPTER V

Losing It All

After our trip from knowing where our heads would rest to not knowing where our next meal would come from, we were exhausted. Tim had done all the driving for four days and I was sore from riding. We weren't sure yet where we would end up, but we were at a stopping place for right now. We would do a little visiting and have, for the next couple of days, a place to take a shower.

One evening, Tim and I were discussing the unresolved compassionate reassignment issue and thought of SGT Cooper from CCAD. She was the clerk there that had been so sweet in helping us. She had been reassigned. Her situation was about not wanting the duty station she had been assigned to. While SGT Cooper had been overseas, her mother had been taking care of her daughter. Now her mother was not doing well and needed SGT Cooper to take care of her and the granddaughter. The military fought her on a compassionate reassignment, but she had persisted and won. She ended up at CCAD because this was the duty station closest to her mother. In the process, SGT Cooper decided to apply for (and received) a discharge. She had had enough of the military telling her what was more vital and sending her away from who she considered most important in her life. Way to go SGT Cooper! You stood up for yourself and won the right to live and think on your own.

How we hoped our outcome would be the same. Somehow, we knew it wouldn't. I had caused to many problems for the military. They had lost face during the South Korean accident and I was at the base of why the outcome there changed. The military wanted to see us in a gutter before they would do the right thing.

Two more compassionate reassignments have come to our attention. These made national newspapers and made us see that compassionate reassignments could be granted. Lyme Disease and a dying wife were just not the reasons for allowing one for Tim.

The first one is a reservist with an active duty husband serving in Iraq. It happened in Denver, Colorado in November 2003. The newspaper said "Simone Holcomb was a soldier motivated by duty and honor who knew the sacrifices her job required and performed without complaint". This was no different than what Tim had done for over twenty years. He had served without any complaints, and his duty and honor were above reproach. When I was dying, his duty and honor came in the form of saving my life. But the U.S. Army wouldn't have that! He was told by PERSCOM that the "Korea tour had priority over family issues". This meant that the military didn't care if I lived or died, just so Tim was back in South Korea to pass out drivers' licenses.

The article said that Simone Holcomb chose her children over the military when she was forced into a corner. This was over a custody battle (her husband's children) and the lack of someone to care for the children while they were away. Their family care plan had failed and they were left with little choice. We can all understand this, I am sure. There was no life and death situation the military had to consider. This could have possibly been cleared up with an extension of time, as we have seen other similar situations straightened out. Instead, the military was trying to lump this soldier into the pot of all the other soldiers who had come home on leave and never returned. In the end, this soldier who had served seven years was granted a compassionate reassignment. Hooah!

Tim had not come home on leave and was enjoying himself so much that he just didn't want to return to South Korea. In fact, he was actually enjoying the tour and even promised to bring back a tea set when he came home at the end of the tour. He liked the low profile job the military had to hide him in and he was looking forward to ending the long career with a clean record. This mid-tour leave was to take care of my medical needs and hurry back to South Korea. It didn't roll that way. I thank God for giving my husband a good brain and the strength to do the right thing. Without Tim, I would surely have died. Would the military be there for my husband then? No.

The reason I say "no" is due to a conversation I overheard at the Personnel Office at Ft. Sam Houston one after noon while waiting for copies of orders. The conversation was between the CSM and a chaplain about a memorial service for a soldier that had been killed in Iraq. The two were joking about the soldier's father and mother who were divorced. The father wanted to be recognized at the memorial service and the mother was not comfortable with this. They were actually making a joke of this soldier's parents disagreement. The two men were also saying what an inconvenience it was to have this memorial service, what with all the security and big deal this was causing. I was disgusted with this banter, but there was no place for me to go to get out of hearing range. Apparently the two men were not concerned with anyone overhearing their dialogue because the door was left open and voices were not hushed. I was suddenly not very proud of these two soldiers and could almost picture them at the service with their phony smiles and tribute. This soldier gave his life so these two men could sit in an office and make fun of his family and be annoyed that they had to attend his memorial service. One of these men would be the reason one of the compassionate reassignment packets never reached PERSCOM. He chose not to send it.

So, I don't believe that the military would have shown my soldier much sympathy if he had gone back to South Korea and I had died from the 100% intestinal blockage. All because the military decided that this was elective surgery, they refused to allow my husband to be compassionately reassigned. Hell, even when Tim had a leave form with another twenty-one days, the South Korean command still listed him as AWOL and PERSCOM looked the other way. Even the Secretary of the Army and The White House looked the other way. They all knew and they all chose to ignore the chance to do the right thing.

The other compassionate reassignment has to do with a soldier serving in Iraq with a small child and a pregnant wife back in the states. This couple had signed a lease with an option to buy.

However, the lease was up and the option to buy would expire at the end of November, 2003. According to the newspaper report, the soldier had come back for a short two-week leave in mid November 2003 and returned to Iraq. Shortly after his return, the wife was up in arms because she was facing eviction. The post rushed to help her and the last we read, the soldier was being considered for a compassionate reassignment. This was not a compassionate reassignment he was asking for, but with the headlines, it was offered.

So, if I had been asking for a compassionate reassignment because I was being evicted, would we had had a better chance? If we had had a child care issue, would there have been a newspaper story done and a compassionate reassignment authorized? We seriously doubt it. These soldiers were not in South Korea where rules and regulations are there on paper but can be erased or altered by the stroke of a pen to suit a command. Like the stroke of the pen that listed Tim illegally AWOL. Did the Pentagon know? Yes. Did The White House know? You bet. Did anyone care? Not on your life.

While Tim was in South Korea and putting in the paperwork for the first compassionate reassignment, he learned of a Chaplain who was being granted a curtailment. This soldier had been in South Korea for almost a year, but shy of his tour. The Chaplain's wife who was back in the states and had been diagnosed with some form of mild cancer. Based on her diagnosis, the curtailment was granted and he was reassigned back in the states to take care of his wife.

The first couple of days in our new location, we decided that we didn't have enough money to go anywhere else. We were stuck here and needed a place to live. A smaller than small apartment was for rent and for six hundred dollars, we could move in. We had only a little over that amount, but we were forced to take it. We would deal with food and gasoline as best we could.

The next challenge we had was furniture. If we bought groceries and put gasoline in our vehicle, we could not buy furniture. Instead, we went dumpster-diving, visited garage sales and borrowed from a relative. The apartment was not fancy, but we were thrilled to be out of the weather.

Tim knew he had to find a job. With no income, we would be evicted as we had been in Texas. In this area, there are very few jobs available, but God was looking out for us. He was able to get a job within two weeks and it even offered insurance for a fee. The hours were long and the work very unfamiliar to Tim, but he would do anything to keep food on the table. From the U.S. Army to The White House, they had all let us down. I was sure thankful I had a brave and honorable soldier looking out for me. I never felt safer. My husband was suddenly my hero and I was his fan club. We now knew what "The Army of One" was all about.

After 9/11, I learned that NIS now fell under Homeland Security. This should have made me feel more safe, but after reading a report that The Wall Street Journal (WSJ) put out on April 25, 2003, I was not sure that "safe" was the word I would use. While living in Texas, it was not uncommon to be living among illegal aliens. Heck, I knew they were there. Almost everyone knew they were living and working there.

The WSJ's report stated that when the government decides to deport a foreigner, they send a "bag and baggage letter" to the one to be deported. Nothing like giving the foreigner a head start.

It was reported that 355,000 had been issued this letter over the years. With the tightened security in 2002, it said that our government decided to hunt for these foreigners. Agents rounded up 2,256 absconders and 696 of those have been deported. In 1996, the files that contain every name of these foreigners were being held in Vermont. In that same year, the immigration authorities budgeted $11 million for 142 clerks to enter these foreigners' names into the national crime database. The clerks were not hired and no word on where the money went. Now, it will take until 2006 to get the names entered into the database, as the report goes.

But of course, before the clerks are hired, they will have to have a background check. Then, the government will probably only hire a dozen clerks to enter the names. With the coffee breaks and lunches, these clerks will probably have about five and a half hours of productive time at their desks. Figure in that they will probably be people who will want to have job security, so maybe twenty names will be entered into the database per day. Then, the government will need to take money from that project so they can spend the money on writing up new rules and regulations that can be bent and broken if it serves the purpose of the military. My guess, by the year 2020, the job of entering names of foreigners into the database may get done. Yes, makes me feel safe.

In 2003, Homeland Security spent nearly fifty-six billion dollars. Paying an Army Surgeon General to show any form of compassion would definitely get my vote on the budget. Or paying someone to find missing medical records; education for military physicians with regards to Lyme Disease; or returning Tim's stuff back from the South Korean command. These would all be good things to do with some of that government budget.

I sent a certified letter to the South Korean command in December, 2003, with a copy to The Department of The Army. Since Tim had walked many soldiers through the AWOL and DFR (Dropped From Rolls) process, I knew that getting Tim's personal belongings back was something I was entitled to, being his next of kin. However, after almost three months, I have not heard a word. That regulation is just another one they have seen fit to break. It's not like we can replace some of the items still supposedly stored in South Korea. Nothing takes the place of your own possessions. Pictures, television, DVD player, clothes, and more. They have not only reduced us to poverty, as far as I can tell, they have stolen my husband's belongings. And The Department of The Army is ignoring this, as well.

Tim thought of applying for a Chapter 6 Hardship Discharge or putting in his retirement paperwork (it was well within the time frame to do so). However, due to the Stop-Loss (no one gets out or retires), it left him no other option than to stand and fight. This is what a soldier is trained to do anyway. We just didn't think Tim would have to be fighting his own branch of the military. We even inquired about an attorney. But fifteen thousand dollars is more than we have, even IF Guy Womack said that he was confident that he could get Tim his retirement. For a financially strapped soldier and his wife, it becomes a waiting game. We wait for the military to do the right thing and the military waits for us to give up.

I won't give up. Have you heard of the "war on drugs"; "war on terrorism"; and the "war on poverty"? I would like to declare a "war on indifference". My weapons are my stamina and belief in doing the right thing. This book is the product of that determination and conviction. With this book, I hope to end the U.S. Army's unresponsiveness; wipe out their lack of compassion; bring to an end to their coldness; terminate their lack of sympathy; put a stop to their apathy; and stop their lack of concern. The U.S. Army's total lack of interest in helping Tim save my life is unacceptable. Their laziness in handling this situation is sickening. Their estimation of my fortitude is infuriating.

CHAPTER VI

Life In Purgatory

After Tim started working and the insurance kicked in, I started looking for a doctor who would be able to treat my Lyme Disease. It was not going to be an easy task. It hadn't been so far.

The first doctor's office I called said that they would treat Lyme Disease, but never had before. The doctor would be willing to work with me, so reported the receptionist. Being an Internist, I thought I would be in good hands again and hopefully get the IV therapy I desperately needed. Besides, this was the very same physician that had treated my daughter-in-law when she had cancer a couple years ago. She passed away, but it had nothing to do with the doctor. She was a very sick young lady with a cancer that only infects the elderly. It is so rare in anyone young that my daughter-in-law was written up in a medical journal. However, there was no cure and was not being studied. Sounds a little like the Lyme Disease situation.

I made the appointment and remembered to bring my medical records for his review. Tim accompanied me to the exam room. As always, it was easier for him to let the doctor know if I had missed something that I ought to tell him. Or if I had trouble finding words, Tim knew the story as well as I did.

The physician was pleasant but appeared suddenly to be an

expert on Lyme Disease. When I offered him brochures, he rejected them. He said that he knew all about this disease. I was suspicious. But I was a good sport and since this was already costing us, I would make the most of the office visit.

I explained that I was there basically to renew prescriptions for my medications (one I had been out of for almost three months and the others would soon be gone). He examined me on the table and commented that I had dry skin. I told him that no amount of lotion could counteract the chemicals in the water here. He went on to tell me that my joints were swollen and asked if I had any pain. Okay, now suspicion was definitely the way to go here. Anyone who has Lyme Disease knows that joint swelling and pain are common symptoms.

The exam ended with the doctor asking for a drug test. I agreed to the test as I believed he wanted to rule out "drug user" as a diagnosis. One of the prescriptions I needed was Ultracet, a mild pain reliever.

A few days after this visit, I received a certified letter from the doctor. It stated that he could no longer treat me as I had not been truthful with him. He had found no Ultracet in my lab results. Therefore, the doctor-patient relationship would not work.

I was furious. I had not only explained that I had been out of this medication for almost three months, but it was in my medical records when the last refill had been, and the drug was on my medication list that he copied. I called his office, but he would not speak with me. His nurse said that she remembered why I had been there (medication refills), but did not know about the letter from the doctor that I was referring to.

I wrote this doctor a letter, sent it certified and decided to send a copy of both letters to the government agencies that oversee physicians here.

He just didn't listen or have empathy for me. Could it be that mistakes are made in the medical field so often because some doctors have the 'know it all' attitude? I believe this has a great deal to do with the blunders made. Reporting this doctor was something I felt needed doing. He may have gotten away with this in the past, but with a statement on file, I hoped someone would now be monitoring.

I had my medications, but it was time to find another physician. I did one of the best things I could do for myself. I joined an Internet support group for people who had Lyme Disease, also known as Lymers or Lymies. I found that there are thousands of Lymers and almost as many who are concerned for a Lymer.

Some of the stories broke my heart more than others. Even with what Tim and I were going through, I still had room in my heart to show compassion for other Lymers and their families.

Poor Pamela couldn't afford anymore treatments. She could not work and even though she had applied for Social Security Disability, it would be two years before she received any help, if she were even approved.

Roger was new to treatments and was worried about the reactions he was experiencing after being put on antibiotics. He was scared that living with Lyme Disease may not be as bad as having a "herx".

A Herxheimer reaction is, nicknamed "herx", or better known as Jarisch-Herxheimer. It is a reaction that has been observed when treating Syphilis but has been witnessed with other illnesses as well(Lyme Disease 1991-Patient/Physician Perspectives from the U.S. and Canada The Jarisch-Herxheimer Reaction, James H. Katzel, MD). In laymen terms, it describes the increase of symptoms when taking antibiotics.

Both Lyme Disease and Syphilis are caused by a bacteria known as a spirochete (pronounced Spear-o-keet). Lyme Disease is caused by a Borrelia burgdorferi and Syphilis, by a Treponema pallidum. Both are spirochetes.

It is believed that when antibiotics are taken for Lyme Disease, the medication causes the toxins within the spirochete to be released in our bodies as they are broken down or killed. This causes a reaction to the toxins and most of the time, not to the antibiotics (better to check with your physician to make sure if it's a herx or a true allergic reaction). With this herx, Lyme Disease symptoms increase and new symptoms may appear. Some common symptoms are increased joint or muscle pain, headaches, chills, fever, hypotension, hives or a rash, yeast infections among others. There does not seem to be any timing, frequency, or duration consistencies in regards to a herx. Some Lymers experience a herx within days to weeks, if at all. Sometimes it happens once or twice, while others experience a herx throughout the entire therapy. The good news for

Roger is that it looks like herxing is a sign of the antibiotics working, but he's checking with his doctor.

Elaine is new to the group and worried about her 78-year old mother. Seems "Mom" was diagnosed, treated, and released, but is having difficulty sleeping, problems with her memory, is always tired, and complains of living in a fog. Elaine cannot seem to locate a doctor that will take her mother's complaints seriously.

June reports that during a herx, she says that she wanted to find the biggest 18-wheeler and jump in front of it.

Patty says she knows it's discouraging to have a herx, but her doc told her to suffer with it as long as she could. It was actually a good sign. Her advice to Roger was, "don't let it get the best of you. Life is challenging when you look healthy but feel like crap inside. People just think you're complaining. So it's important to have a group of people that can relate to what you're going through".

If we can't convince physicians that we are very ill, how are we supposed to persuade others to believe us? Could it be the fear of prosecution over treating Lyme Disease that we cannot get the doctors to cooperate?

It is not a secret that many kind, caring physicians who chose to take their oath seriously, are being chased down like criminals and prosecuted for treating Lyme Disease. Some have already lost their licenses and their livelihoods. In most cases, it was not because they refused to treat or ignored the patients' complaints. It was due to the governing organizations wanting the doctors to play ball according to their rules. Even though we all know that each patient is different and responds to therapy differently, the powers that be wanted a standard treatment protocol that would treat each patient the same. Unlike Cancer treatment, where different treatments and durations are in order, Lyme Disease was treated as though it were a common cold. Ten to thirty days of antibiotics were what everyone should follow, so said the powers that rule. No matter that this plan did not work for second and third stage Lyme Disease patients.

This is a fragment of what another list member thinks:

Physicians of mainstream medicine are afraid of Lyme Disease or rather treating anyone who has it due to the fear of prosecution from the powers that be for fraud. In as much as there is no definitive test for Lyme Disease, the clinical diagnosis rests with them. Doctors don't want to lose their livelihood and I don't blame them, but doing nothing is the same as causing harm. Instead, they (some doctors) put stuff in our records that defame us and call us difficult patients. They hide behind inadequate testing methodology so they don't have to treat us. Considering the ability of the spirochete to change its protein structure and thereby evading detection, the chances of getting a positive serum test is almost impossible. Politicians declare Lyme Disease in their states is not a problem. They would have to deal with a decline in tourism and address responsibilities they are entrusted with concerning their citizens. It's theorized that pharmaceutical companies are in it for the money. It was written by this list member that if everyone would test positive for the h-pylori and received the 14-day antibiotic, heartburn would be wiped out. Then what would happen to the pockets of the drug barons? Even the PGA is reluctant to speak out about Lyme Disease (a couple of pro-golfers seem to have LD). The PGA could not very well sell tickets and have people out on the course, next to woods. They would surely lose money.

Key words are used when describing Lymers like hypochondriac, delusional, obsessive, compulsive, manic, depressive, psychosomatic, among others. Most of us have been tested for or misdiagnosed with post traumatic stress disorder, bipolar, Multiple Sclerosis, ALS, fibromyalgia, migraines, sleep apnea due to flee or flight innate mental response, raynauds syndrome (a circulatory problem that periodically triggers spasms in the blood vessels of the fingers and toes), degenerative joint disease, post polio syndrome, peripheral neuropathy (describes damage to the peripheral nerves, the vast communications network that transmits information from the brain and spinal cord to every other part of the body-such as with Carpal Tunnel Syndrome), connective tissue disease such as Lupus, ankylosing sodalities (a painful, progressive, rheumatic disease. It mainly affects the spine but it can also affect other joints, tendons and ligaments. Other areas, such as the eyes, lungs, bowel and heart can also be involved), and more.

Amy writes that she is 45 years old and has all the symptoms of Lyme Disease since 1976. It took her twenty-seven years to find a doctor and get the diagnosis of Lyme Disease. She is a computer technician and says that her brain fog is so thick sometimes that she forgets whatever she knew about computers. She says that her memory is poor, too. She can recall childhood, but could not tell you what she did just yesterday.

Kerry states that she has problems with her eyes. She used to be an avid reader and can now not read if the type is on a white background. She suffers severe migraines and is unable to work with all the other symptoms of Lyme Disease. She says she has gained so much weight and now has difficulties walking or sitting for long periods of time. Her thyroid tests keep coming back negative, as do other tests ruling out additional diseases.

Another woman, Marlene, says that she was paralyzed from the neck down and suffering from Lyme Disease symptoms. She took antibiotics (abx) for over five years and used to advocate for them. Now, she says she believes that the medication just chases the bacteria in hopes of catching it, but this never happens. Now, she detoxes her body, cleanses it, nourishes it, and rebuilds it. Her words. She says she is using Artemesinin and claims it works well for cancer and malaria, too. Then, she says she uses a natural antibiotic (Cat's Claw). She ends saying that it has permanent results. (I could never get her to pin down the statistics or get any further information from her).

Julian says that her insurance company paid for three months of IV antibiotic treatment after she was diagnosed. The insurance company decided she was cured and refused to pay for anymore therapy. Now, each time she needs tests, medicine or another doctor, she must go through many, many appeals.

Maggie thinks that there's one thing that doctors "don't get". She believes that a low sugar, plant-centered diet is part of the maintenance program. Doctors, in her opinion, are not health experts since they miss this important part of good heath. Sounds like she believes that eating healthy is the key.

Betty says she would "sell the house" to get on IV antibiotic therapy. She has been suffering with Lyme Disease for seven years and her MRIs have come back twice with lesions (common in acute Lyme patients). She states that she is amazed at how little doctors know about this disease or how misinformed they are.

Nellie has just been tested and is waiting for the results from Igenex Laboratory in California. Says she that she is pretty sure she has the disease, but could use some encouragement. The symptoms are overwhelming.

Lydia says that her mother has Lyme Disease and sees an internist. He does not treat the 81 year old woman (who still lives alone and drives only in her own neighborhood). The doctor just pats her hand and tells her she is doing well.

In the Philly Inquirer, staff reporter writes on January 20, 2004 that "Walter S. 'Terry' Batty, Jr. is retiring after 32 years as the U.S. attorney's first career prosecutor and first appeals chief from a debilitating back injury aggravated by long-term Lyme Disease." Batty was interviewed over the telephone and said that it was impossible for him to even come to work and retirement was "unavoidable".

Other patients on the list have noted slurred speech, numbness in toes and fingers, lost cognitive and motor skills, among other symptoms.

A doctor friend of mine has Lyme Disease. She is a sweetheart and having such a rough time. She had a thriving practice and was self-medicating for her Lyme Disease. The other physicians in her area did not believe Lyme Disease was a concern and accused her of being "on drugs". She went before the medical review board and they gave her no other choice than to check herself in to a clinic for a week (at her own expense) and be tested for drug and alcohol abuse.

The results came back that she was not an abuser, but this was not enough for her peers. She still slurred her speech and found it difficult to find words at times. The board now knew she was not an abuser, but they did not believe she had Lyme Disease. She was then to go to their choice of a physician to be tested for Lyme Disease. Not a Lyme Literate Physician, but one that was from their jar of doctors. This was a nightmare for this woman of medicine. She had done nothing wrong. She was only guilty of struggling with this debilitating disease while trying to treat patients. She gives her medical opinion online free to those of us who need it. She explains the tests, diagnosis, and treatments, in a way we all can understand. When there is a question that needs an answer, she is more than willing to answer. She knows what it is to be abused by the very people who took an oath not to do any harm. She is fighting her own (the doctors) just as Tim is fighting his own (the military).

CHAPTER VII

Life and Death With Lyme Disease

In The Quad City Times Newspaper, Iowa journalist Cheri Black writes an article titled "Doctor Shares Experiences About Lyme Disease". The doctor is Scott Taylor and he says that he "doesn't know when or where he was bitten by a tick that caused him to contract Lyme Disease. His symptoms were subtle and spanned nearly three years, including ringing in his ears, changes in his heart rhythm, insomnia, dizziness and muscle twitches."

He had to visit many different physicians and had to undergo several tests for other diseases before he found a physician in Springfield, Illinois who "finally diagnosed Lyme Disease."

Since his diagnoses, Dr. Taylor began researching this disease and now "lectures about his findings to physicians, sufferers of the disease and people just wanting to learn more." Dr. Taylor also went on to say that he believes this disease is "underreported, misdiagnosed, and more prevalent than anyone is aware of."

In another article by Liz Babiarz of The Fredericks News-Post, another doctor made news. In 2001, his patient was suffering and no one could figure out how to treat his ailments. The patient suffered with double vision, high blood pressure, fatigue, and shortness of breath. He started losing weight, developed Bell's Palsy (facial paralysis), had difficulty swallowing, his equilibrium was off, and he had severe neck stiffness. Even after numerous visits with five specialists, no one found the cause.

The patient stated that "more and more things kept happening until one morning, he woke up and was unable to swallow his own saliva". After a trip to the local hospital, he was diagnosed with Lou Gehrig's Disease and given six months to live. He was sent home on a feeding tube and wanted to die.

The patient's friend told him about a man who died from what doctors thought was Lou Gehrig's Disease but turned out to be Lyme Disease. The patient made an appointment with Dr. Gregory Bach, a Philadelphia-born physician. After six months, the patient was feeling more like his old self. After nine months, he reported that most of the symptoms had vanished. Dr. Bach was quoted as saying that he wanted the ELISA test removed from the market because it was not reliable.

Dr. John Drulle was 59 years old and had suffered from Lyme Disease for over fifteen years. He passed away on November 7, 2003. He is sorely missed and not just because he was a first-class Lyme Literate physician, but he was also a wonderful educator and family man. He was a friend to many and in the Lyme Disease community, a comrade is gold.

Suicide never crossed my mind until I started developing my many symptoms with Lyme Disease. I had no
Plan to make my passing easier, but I thought that if I could just lay down and stop breathing, all my troubles would be over. No more pain. What a blessing this would be for me. I feel such sorrow for the family members left behind when their loved one dies. But, I am torn because I feel such joy that the person who was in so much pain and agony has finally a release from the shackles of a disease. Though pain became routine to my everyday life, something keeps driving me to live. I am not sure if it is the hope of a cure or the need to help others with this horrible disease, but there's a reason that I am still alive.

"ACE Recipient's Passing", were headlines on Monday, December 08, 2003 in Pennsylvania. The first paragraph said it all. "We are deeply sorry to announce that the 2003 ACE Award winner in the Search and Rescue Category, Pepper, a German Shepherd Dog, died recently from complications from Lyme Disease. We extend our condolences to Richard and

Myrna Goodwin of Croydon, Pennsylvania."

Not only does Lyme Disease take human lives, it takes man's best friends.

There was a thread started about the sense of dying. Before Lyme Disease, I never felt like I was dying. Why should I? I was always healthy as the proverbial horse.

When the question was posed, there were many responses. I learned that this, among other sensitive topics, was difficult to describe. Just knowing that we are not alone with this disease and all of its symptoms I believe, makes us stronger.

Some of the following is other Lymers' experience with this sense of dying. It is not as uncommon as we would like to imagine.

*When I was very ill I felt as though I hovered between life and death, and that I was, really, more dead than alive. I think when you are in a lot of pain the spirit moves away from the body and certainly I had many strange dreams and half waking half dreaming hallucinations. I suppose some of it might be a kind of sensory deprivation like a flotation chamber. But I'm not afraid of dying now. Writing about this has made me feel less alone."

*I have been also exactly like this before. I am not like this now (thank God) but I at times still have that nagging fear that it is all going to came back. After improving to this point I have not experienced this total involvement with the dread, depression, isolation and negativity that Lyme causes - along with the physical symptoms on top of it. This is one aspect of this insane disease - it is such an all inclusive attack that it overwhelms us. We are still in there somewhere - at the deepest level of ourselves we are still "alive" and of course on "good days" we can feel that we are still "there".

*I don't think it matters on or off the medication as far as feeling that sense of dying. At least not for me."

*This sense of dying... I know what you speak about. I think it is 'dying' in many ways. There is so much physical exhaustion, mental exhaustion, emotional exhaustion, and spiritual exhaustion that is wrapped up in Lyme Disease. It is so taxing. It attacks one's life in all directions and leaves the person's body and soul so brutally beaten that how can one not have that sense of dying?"

*I get out of bed everyday, drag myself to work so I at least have insurance, no matter how much my body hurts, and somehow

I do make it through the day holding on by a string, and drop with total exhaustion when I get home. I'm glad to know that other people have this looming sense of dying over them. It's overwhelming."

*That's exactly the feeling I've had all the years I've had Lyme. I've described it to several doctors and they and each send me to a different specialist. And of course, they all wanted to give me the Anti-Depressant dejour.. Until I saw this post just now, I never knew anyone else had this sensation... "

*This 'Sense of Dying' I am referring to is not the same as a depressive episode. Most times it occurs after laying down for a nap or to sleep - usually a "herx", or "crash" precedes. I tend to go over a short list of uncompleted tasks, right before going into a comatose-like state, which results in a very deep sleep. I guess the physical sensation is similar to feeling anesthetized, but the feeling or thoughts or knowingness lends itself to coming to a place of surrender and acceptance that you are passing over, and all struggle ceases. It is not alarming, nor anxious ... in fact it is a very peaceful state. But there is a definite knowingness that you are crossing over. I know I feel surprised to still be alive. Which is very different than wanting to die, or wishing to be dead."

My own sense of dying was the strangest experience I have ever had. It happened one evening at bedtime. Nothing out of the ordinary happened during the day; no mysterious new symptoms; and meals were as usual. I was in no more pain than I was accustomed to and only had a light Lyme Fog.

I got ready for bed and slipped under the blankets. I put my CPAP mask on, turned on the machine, and rested my head on my pillow. I closed my eyes, but within minutes, an odd sensation came over me.

I was feeling such peace. The impression I remember was lighter than air, but not floating; beautiful surroundings but being nowhere; and not wanting to leave this amazing freedom.

I recall feeling that I had taken care of everything I needed to (will, letters, etc.) and there was no need to do anything except stay "at this time" forever.

I was not asleep because I heard the street traffic. It wasn't as loud as usual, but the vehicles were real. I felt the air from my CPAP, but it no longer stung my eyes.

The following morning, I was almost euphoric, but with a sense of despair. I was overjoyed that I could recall the space I had been in, but despair because I was still alive, to struggle another day. That morning, I felt I had been given a preview of dying.

I have never been afraid to die. However, I am now looking forward to God's call home.

This portion of an article appeared on August 24,1993 in The New York Times. The reporter was Elisabeth Rosenthal.
"From her bed at Northern Westchester Hospital Center,
Vicki Logan begs to differ with academic scientists who claim that there is no such thing as chronic Lyme infection and that Lyme is cured with at most four weeks of antibiotics.

Since 1987, Ms. Logan has battled headaches, fevers, fatigue, progressive paralysis, seizures, periods of dementia and memory loss so severe that she remembers only the previous three weeks out of the last year. For much of her illness doctors told her she could not possibly have Lyme Disease and prescribed no antibiotics.

Two years ago Dr. Kenneth Liegner, a Westchester internist, decided to buck conventional wisdom and try giving her prolonged courses of antibiotics that could kill the Lyme spirochete: She improved somewhat during each course of the drugs, and relapsed when they were stopped. Dr. Liegner became convinced that Ms. Logan had chronic
active Lyme infection that could be controlled but not cured through daily drug treatment.

Others, including consultants at the Mayo Clinic, disputed the diagnosis, saying that after months of antibiotics, Ms. Logan -- if she ever had Lyme -- had certainly been cured. But recently, Dr. Liegner was vindicated: scientists at the Centers for Disease Control and Prevention in Atlanta found the Lyme spirochete, Borrelia burgdorferi, swimming in a sample of Ms. Logan's spinal fluid.

"My life prior to the last three weeks is a blank," Ms. Logan said in a halting voice. "I've lost everything and I'll be going to a nursing home when I get out of the hospital. If you think you have Lyme disease, you have to pursue the diagnosis."

A handful of cases like Ms. Logan's are challenging conventional assumptions about Lyme disease and igniting a fiery debate about the usual course of this increasingly common infection: Are disastrous experiences with Lyme like hers the rare exception or the rule?

Most people who are treated shortly after a tick bite tend to recover uneventfully, but a small number go on to develop chronic symptoms which they attribute to Lyme infection despite extensive antibiotic treatment. These patients, who sometimes receive months of home intravenous treatments and experience serious disability, account for
the lion's share of the health care dollars spent on the illness. They fill the growing number of Lyme support groups.

And yet doctors are unsure which, if any, of them actually has active Lyme. Many of the country's leading Lyme experts believe that the number is microscopic. "I think persistent infection occurs but it is very, very rare," said Dr. John J. Halperin, professor of neurology at North Shore University Hospital on Long Island. "There are a lot
of people being labeled chronic Lyme with very little evidence of it. They don't have Lyme and so they won't respond to a zillion months of antibiotics." Some of the patients' complaints -- generally fatigue, joint aches and cognitive problems -- may be due to permanent tissue damage from Lyme sustained before antibiotic treatment, Dr. Halperin said, or to some poorly defined immune
reaction set off by prior infection. He and many other doctors say they believe that the majority never had Lyme at all.

On the other side are Dr. Liegner and other doctors who say their practices are filled with Lyme patients who do not get better. They say academic experts are so blinded by what they "know" that they cannot see the evidence piling up in front of their eyes.

"I think that Lyme is an incurable disease in many patients -- there's no question in my mind about that -- and I think that's being suppressed and denied," Dr. Liegner said. "Cases like Vicki Logan's are not exceptions; they reveal the problems with our current paradigm."

Vickie Logan's insurance company refused to pay for long-term care. She passed away on July 17, 2003, still praying for treatment or a cure.

There are plenty of people who believe that Lyme Disease is curable after short-term antibiotics. In some cases, the disease moves from early to late stage and sometimes to death. I just wonder when we will have the medical community on one sheet of music. This Lyme dance cannot continue with so many tunes playing. We have already seen some of the marathoners dropping out. We don't seem to be any closer today than we were thirty years ago of making this disease noteworthy, treatable on an individual patient regime, or a cure. We don't even be able to get a handful of physicians to agree that there is Chronic Lyme Disease. Could there be more to this than just a simple case of disagreeing on treatment protocol or believing that Lyme Disease exists at all?

I recently learned that a woman was allowed to die with Lyme Disease. Her husband didn't believe the disease existed and refused to seek treatment for his wife. I was so sad that this woman had to suffer with this disease, but even worse, she did it alone.

CHAPTER VIII

Who Knows About Lyme Disease?

The Girl Scouts know that Lyme Disease exists. They have a "Tickbuster Patch Program" that increases awareness and prevention of Lyme Disease. (For more information on this course, the American Lyme Disease Foundation asks you to call them at 914-934-8860). The girls learn all about ticks and ways to protect themselves.

The Boy Scouts do not have a patch program, but in 2001, they were having cards printed up for their Scout Jamboree. One side of the card is about tick bite prevention. The reverse side deals with spiders and venomous insects.

What about The Center for Disease Control (CDC)? Surely they should know something about this disease. They have been collecting data on reported cases since 1982. I was curious so I visited their website. This would prove to be my first step into the Whos, Whats and Wheres of Lyme Disease.

The first thing I wanted to know was how many reports of Lyme Disease were collected. From 1982 through 2001, I added up 190,518. CDC suggests that this number multiplied by ten percent is a more accurate figure. They know it is underreported at least by this proportion. That leaves us with 1,905,180(-+) people who have Lyme Disease through 2001. On the same website, there was a separate division for HIV/AIDS prevention. It stated there was, to date, reports of 886,575 cases. And since Cancer is also making the news, I checked with The National Cancer Institute's website. There, I learned that in 2003, they were estimating that there would be 1,334,199 new cases. CDC lists Arthritis, Cancer, Diabetes, Epilepsy and Heart Disease as "chronic diseases". Nowhere did I find Lyme Disease listed as a chronic disease.

How does a Lyme Disease case get to CDC's statistic statement? The latest information on this question was posted to the CDC website in 1996. Clinical description is "a systemic, tick borne disease with protein manifestations, including dermatologic (skin), rheumatologic (arthritis), neurologic (brain), and cardiac abnormalities. The best clinical marker for the disease is the initial skin lesion
(Erythema migrans {EM}) that occurs in 60-80% of patients. Okay, this says to me that Lyme Disease can be clinically diagnosed. But, the report went on to define CDC's reporting criteria for making the surveillance list. "Laboratory criteria for diagnosis is 1) Isolation of Bb (Lyme Disease) from clinical specimen or, 2) demonstration of diagnostic immunoglobulin M or G antibodies to Bb in serum (blood) or cerebrospinal fluid (CSF). A two-test approach using a sensitive ELISA followed by a Western blot is recommended."

This would be a spinal tap or a two-part serum test. An ELISA titer (not sensitive, according to many physicians) and Western blot (if the titer was positive).

Now, if Arthritis is listed as a chronic disease and Lyme Disease has manifestations that include arthritis, why isn't Lyme Disease listed under chronic diseases? And, if the titer test is not sensitive to detect Lyme Disease, then why is it part of CDC's criteria? Finally, if Lyme Disease can be clinically diagnosed (the CDC lists was to look for when clinically diagnosing), then why doesn't CDC accept clinical diagnosis of the disease? I was finding myself asking more questions than discovering answers.

On the same CDC site, I found a list posted showing the leading causes of disabilities. Arthritis was number one. It said that 7 out of every 10 Americans die each year due to chronic diseases; 25 million people have major limitations due to chronic diseases; 90 million people live with chronic diseases; and 75% of our nation's $1.4 Trillion is spent in medical costs due to chronic diseases.

CDC states, under Lyme Disease symptoms, "infection in the

untreated or inadequately treated patient may progress to late disseminated disease weeks to months after infection. The most common objective manifestation of late disseminated Lyme disease is intermittent swelling and pain of one or a few joints, usually large, weight-bearing joints such as the knee. Some patients develop chronic axonal polyneuropathy, or encephalopathy, the latter usually manifested by cognitive disorders, sleep disturbance, fatigue, and personality changes. Infrequently, Lyme disease morbidity may be severe, **chronic**, and disabling. An ill-defined post-Lyme disease syndrome occurs in some persons following treatment for Lyme disease. Lyme disease is rarely, if ever, fatal."

Now, I was confused. At the CDC site, Lyme Disease was not listed under "chronic diseases", but it clearly states that Lyme Disease may very well be "chronic". If the titer test was not sensitive, why bother? If arthritis is part of Lyme Disease and is the number one cause for disabilities, why do people applying for Social Security Disability have so much trouble getting it? And, if 7 out of 10 people die each year from chronic diseases, then why did CDC say that LD was rarely fatal, if ever? Didn't they know about the deaths from Lyme Disease or complications from the disease? The further I researched, the more confusing this dilemma became. But, I was a military wife and knew that if I searched long enough, I would surely come up with answers.

The latest details from The World Health Organization (WHO) was not promising. I could not find much information on their website about Lyme Disease. I sent them an email, addressed to NCD Surveillance (the chronic disease department). The reply was received two days later. It said that they did not cover Lyme Disease in that department. I was referred back to their website, where I found the same lack of information and no studies being conducted. Didn't WHO receive funding to study all diseases in the world? I was sure that I read that somewhere.

Next, I researched the Food and Drug Administration (FDA). Since this was the organization responsible for approving tests and drugs, I wanted to see what good news they were promoting about Lyme Disease.

In the FDA's Article 312.80-Purpose, I found that the FDA "expedites the development, evaluation, and marketing of new therapies intended to treat persons with life-threatening and severely-debilitating illnesses, especially where no satisfactory alternative therapy exists. In Article 312.81-Scope, it states that "life-threatening" means "diseases or conditions where the likelihood of death is high unless the course of the disease is interrupted."

CDC already established that Lyme Disease was debilitating (and anything that lists the brain being affected by a disease, I would be safe in assuming that this would be considered "severe"). Yet, I could find no treatment protocol regarding Lyme Disease. How could this be? Didn't the FDA fund researchers to work on such projects?

This search for answers lead me to the United States Department of Health & Human Services. Here, I found a testimonial statement by Phillip Baker, Ph.D., Lyme Disease Program Officer, Division of Microbiology and Infectious Disease, National Institute of Allergy and Infectious Diseases (NIAD), National Institutes of Health and Human Services. It was titles "Hearing: NIH (National Institute of Health) Lyme Disease Research", dated January 29, 2004. Finally, some current information!

The introduction read, "NIAID has a long-standing commitment to Lyme borreliosis research (Lyme Disease) that began more than 20 years ago when the cause of the disease was not yet known. In 1981, NIAID-funded researchers identified Borrelia burgdorferi as the causative agent of Lyme Disease, and since then, basic and clinical research efforts have been expanded in scope to address a variety of issues, related to this illness. These activities include both intramural and extramural research on animal models, microbial physiology, molecular and cellular mechanisms of pathogeneis, mechanisms of protective immunity, vectors and disease transmissions, efficacy of different modes of antibiotic therapy, and the development of more sensitive and reliable diagnostic tests for both early (acute) and late (chronic) Lyme Disease."

Okay, now we have CDC, the FDA and NIAID stating that there is such a thing as "chronic" Lyme Disease with severe complications, and they are still researching testing diagnostic methods and antibiotic therapy.

It went on to say, "approximately 20% of NIAID's extramural Lyme Disease portfolio is devoted to the development of novel and more sensitive diagnostic procedures; the NIAID also regularly re-evaluates the effectiveness of currently-used diagnostic methods.

In collaboration with the CDC, the Institute plays a major role in the development of new approaches for diagnosing Lyme borreliosis in the presence of co-infecting agents, as well as in individuals who have been immunized."

I understand this to mean that this group apparently know that what is available presently is not sensitive enough. This backs up what the doctors who treat Lyme Disease are saying.

Further reading included that there had been an antibiotic study (New England Medical Center-NEMC, Boston). This study was terminated after 90-days due to "no significant differences in the percentage of patients who felt that their symptoms had improved, worsened, or stayed the same between the antibiotic treatment and the placebo groups in either trial." It went on to state that the NIAID would follow these patients, but no new therapeutic studies would be started until they had the results analyzed. (NEJM 345: 85-93, 2001).

I know that since I have been on antibiotics (1997), I have never felt well, but without them, I cannot function. I didn't need thousands of dollars and a laboratory to figure this out. I believe that not everything is scientific. Some things are just good common sense. If the antibiotics are keeping me from being bedridden, then I will keep taking what works for me and for how ever long I need them. If the medication is not helping or causing other complications, I hope that I have enough brain cells left to make the decision to discontinue the treatment.

In conclusion, it said that NIAID has a comprehensive Lyme Disease research portfolio with the goal of advancing the understanding of the disease and developing ways to improve its diagnosis, treatment, and prevention. The last two lines caught my eye...."In the hope that future research findings will provide important clues to better understanding of this "painful" disease....and, "Lyme Disease research will continue to be a priority for the NIAID for the foreseeable future."

Does this mean that NIAID or their Bethesda-based Laboratory of Clinical Investigation (LCI) is currently working on any Lyme Disease projects?

Dr. Phillip Baker at NIAID, did suggest via email, that I go to ClinicalTrials.gov. I found three clinical trials listed here. The first one listed was an evaluation, treatment, and follow-up. The sponsor was NIAID and included 100 patients. In the summary, the study was being conducted to "learn more about the infection". I did not find a doctor's name in charge of the trial or the date this was to start or end. The second clinical study was titled "Brain Imaging and Retreatment Study of Persistent Lyme Disease", sponsored by NINDS (National Institute of Neurological Disorders and Stroke". There were to be 65 patients involved with Dr. Fallon listed as the physician in charge. Results were expected in February, 2004. The third and final clinical study was titled "Clinical Microbiological and Immunological Characteristics". There were to be 440 patients and the summary described the trial would determine whether the patients who have been treated with antibiotics still have the bacteria and if this bacteria was causing their symptoms. They stated that they hoped to gather information that may lead them to develop a basis for a rigid diagnostic criteria that could be used in future treatment studies. I also noticed that Multiple Sclerosis listed, but could not imagine how this would figure into a Lyme Disease study.

The one word that stood out was "painful". At least NIAID seemed to understand that this disease is indeed that. If they recognized this fact, then why wasn't there more going on to find a relief for our pain?

I would like to say that antibiotics and Motrin have kept my symptoms in check, for the most part since 1997. There have been times when a break was necessary due to the antibiotics no longer working well. But after four days, the symptoms would be severe. I would have to go back on the antibiotics and begin again. I understand that the spirochetes can hide when being bombarded with medications. After medications for so long, I have to assume they find a safe hiding place inside my body. When I stop the medications, they come back out of hiding. It seems like a cycle that cannot be stopped. This is called pulsing the medication.

I next went to the NIH (National Institute of Health). I found that NIH funds the NIAID for infectious disease studies. In 1992, the NIH formed a NIH Lyme Disease Coordinating Committee (LDCC). This committee was created to compliment other agencies interested in such studies. The committee meets annually to review results of studies and gather information of recent advances. The FDA and CDC are included in this information-gathering and have representatives that serve on the LDCC.

On the NIH website, I found what they list as the history of Lyme Disease. In 1975, they state that the first cases of LD are reported; 1989, the outer surface protein (OspA) was found and cloned; early 1990's, OspA was found in many chronic LD patients; 1990-1992, mice were protected with a vaccination (rOspA); 1992-1995, the vaccine was tested in other animals; 1995 Lyme vaccine was safe and effective for people with Lyme Disease; 1995-1998, Lyme vaccine was safe and effective for people without Lyme Disease; and, in 1998, the FDA approved LYMErix that was produced by SmithKline Beecham and the vaccine hit the public in 1999. However, I found a FDA Advisory Committee meeting report (dated January 31, 2001) where Dr. Clare Kahn stated that the vaccine was safe. If the vaccine hit the public in 1999 and a safety meeting was not held until 2001, were they not sure that the vaccine was safe when they produced it for distribution? In nine years, they went from finding and cloning the protein to discovering a vaccine. The vaccine proved to be more dangerous than the disease (causing severe arthritis and actually giving some of the patients the disease). There were about 440,000 people that received the vaccine. One patient stated that she felt like a guinea pig. The vaccine was removed from the market in 2002.

In fact, in 1993, Viera Scheibner, Ph.D. wrote a book titled, "Vaccination: 100 Years of Orthodox Research Shows that Vaccines Represent a Medical Assault on the Immune System". I found that Dr. Scheibner writes that "vaccines are highly noxious", and that vaccines alter the immune system and the immunological response to diseases. In other words, our body's defenses are weakened to ward off diseases.

It is reported that the FDA VAERS (Vaccine Adverse Effects Reporting System) receives about 11,000 reports a year regarding serious adverse reactions with about 1% (112+) resulting in death. It is a federal law that doctors report any deaths due to vaccines, but only a low percentage of physicians actually report.

The NIH Lyme Disease online brochure states that LD is still mistaken for other ailments, is difficult to diagnose, and is "troublesome" to treat in later phases. It also stated that LD does not always respond to treatment.

So, for all the funding that NIH has made to NIAID, all the

information that has been gathered, what advances have been made, if any?

In looking back over the last fifteen years, there doesn't seem to have been many advances. The physicians cannot agree on the treatment protocol. The labs cannot create a sensitive enough test to detect the disease. We see that CDC (whom the medical professionals look to for guidelines), suggest that Lyme Disease cannot be clinically diagnosed (yet, they state what to look for in a clinical diagnosis). And, of course, we have most reporting agencies ignoring the fact that this disease can be fatal. Even if the death was due to a complication to the Lyme Disease, the disease itself is the reason the person died. Common sense. I have seen it stated in newspapers that a person succumbed due to complications of cancer, I can't understand why a person cannot succumb from complications of Lyme Disease. But, I suppose that it may be for the same reason that the majority of the medical profession and the health organizations cannot decide on diagnosis, treatment protocol, or length of therapy. Common sense.

CHAPTER IX

Does Anyone Know About Lyme Disease?

I was sure that I would find some valuable information on The American College of Physician's website. What I found was that they have Lyme Disease diagnosis, treatment, and one statement that made me cringe. It said that Lyme Disease is a curable and preventable disease. Curable?

They list the three stages of Lyme Disease under "diagnosis". With the first stage, fatigue, chills, fever, headaches, joint/muscle pain, swollen lymph nodes, and Erythema Migrans (EMs-bulls eye rash). Second stage lists numbness/pain in arms and legs, paralysis of facial muscles, meningitis (fever, stiff neck and severe headaches), and abnormal heart beats (rare). The third and last stage lists chronic Lyme arthritis, nervous system problems (memory loss and difficulty concentrating), chronic pain in muscles and fitful sleep.

It states that blood tests (titers) alone cannot diagnosis this disease but should be used to confirm. In almost the same breath, they state that ELISA titers and Western blots can produce false positives/negatives. So, how are the tests supposed to confirm anything?

Treatment is listed in two stages, early and late. Early stage is said to be curable with antibiotics while late stage symptoms improve with medications.

So, if I suspect Lyme Disease, I can rely on the symptoms, but not on the blood tests?

Speaking of blood, what happens if I donate blood? Won't I infect others with my tainted blood? It has not been proven that blood from a Lyme Disease victim can cause the disease to be passed on. However, I wondered what the blood banks were doing about screening.

In May of 2003, The American Association of Blood Banks confirmed that there was no useful tests available to screen blood donors, but they require donors to be questioned about any history of babesiosis. If there is a history of this co-infection, the donor is not permitted to donate. Didn't they know that doctors rarely test for co-infections? We have a hard enough time getting tested with unreliable tests, and it's even worse when trying to get tested for a co-infection.

Babesiosis and Ehrilichiosis are co-infections of Lyme Disease. Babesiosis infects the red blood cells. In early signs, fatigue and loss of appetite are common. Later stage may include fever, sweats, muscle aches and headaches. Ehrilichiosis has symptoms that may include fever, myalgia (achy muscles), headaches, leukopenia (a lower number of white cells which causes reduced immune system function), and thrombocytopenia (refers to bleeding that causes bruises or red marks on the skin).

However, if a donor has a history of Lyme Disease, they may donate provided they have taken a full course of antibiotic (and we still don't know what this means as each patient is different) and no longer have symptoms (we know that symptoms may return even after antibiotic treatment).

The American Red Cross says that if the disease is chronic, you cannot donate. If you were treated with antibiotics and completely recovered, you can donate 12 months after the last dose of antibiotics were taken. Again, is there such a thing as complete recovery after being chronic? So far, I haven't found anything to support a complete recovery from chronic Lyme Disease.

The UCSF Blood Centers at Mt. Zion permanently disqualify donors with Lyme Disease. The NY Blood Center says that a donor will be accepted six months after last symptom or 48 hours after treatment and no further symptoms.

In Chicago, paramedics are testing an experimental blood

substitute on severely injured patients (without their consent). This is fairly new and in the experimental stage. So we don't really know for sure if this will work. But we see that the blood banks are not uniform on the Lyme Disease issue, doctors are not all on the same sheet of music and clinical studies seem to be all over the place.

The Johns Hopkins Medical Institution was my next stop. I conversed with the Division of Medical Microbiology and Department of Pathology for answers. I asked if there were currently any studies or trails being conducted or planned in the near future. The response I received stated that they were always trying to put together studies to better understand tick-borne infections, but funding was the issue. Currently, they have no studies that were enrolling patients, but referred me to the NIH and said that this organization had sponsored the best studies to date. With 270 faculty and over 600 research and service personnel, I had hoped that Lyme Disease would be somewhere near the top of their list. But, alas, I was disappointed.

The National Institute of Medicine (NIM) fell next on my list. It was here that I would learn that when someone asks one too many questions, the emails dry up. I asked the agency if there were any studies or trials, as I asked many organizations, and the first response from Jonathon was non-committal. It was vague and never answered my question. I sent another email that was more specific. I knew that in order to get a study done at the NIM, it had to be asked for by a congressman or such. So, I asked if anyone had asked for a study to be done on Lyme Disease and if so, when was it done and where might I find the results.

The response was again vague, but he did say that he knew of no studies that were asked for and had not been done. I took this as, no, no one asked that a Lyme Disease study be done. But, I wanted to clarify this. I sent a third email, but after a month of waiting for a response and none received yet, I doubt this will ever be answered.

I was sure that the military would surely be studying this disease. They had cards and posters, had done a scattered surveillance at installations, and was chemically treating uniforms. I started with The U.S. Army Medical Research Institute of Infectious Diseases in Ft. Detrick, Maryland. This was the Department of Defense's leading laboratory for biological warfare defense (USAMRI-

ID). They were responsible for strategies, information, procedures, and training programs for medical defense against biological threats. They were also contributors with the CDC and WHO. What I found was "nothing". There were no studies. There was no information at all on Lyme Disease.

The next military organization was The National Academy. This is supposed to be "advisors to the nation". I typed in "Lyme Disease", "vector borne", and "tick-borne". These produced no results. However, I was successful when I entered Infectious Disease. I came to four studies. Two were of interest, MFUA-H-99-06-A and BOGH-H-00-01-A. The first one was a review of the DoD Global Emerging Infections Surveillance and Response System (DoD-GEIS). It was started in April of 2000, was to take 18 months and a report would be available October 2001. No report was made available and it looked as though the progress meetings were closed to the public.

The second study was of importance because it was to include CDC, NIH, FDA and others as sponsors. This was supposed to begin May 2001 with the last progress meeting in September 2002. Again, no report was available. I understand that we have to be concerned with national security, but I believe the American citizen is entitled to know if anything was learned. Our tax dollars pay for these studies, but it doesn't appear that we are allowed to have too much information. Reminds me of the parent (U.S. citizens) who works to provide for a thankless, spoiled child.

I personally had more interest in The National Academy as they claim to be the advisors to the nation. This is the organization I see responsible for making sure that the military officers, who are in charge of compassionate reassignments, are kept informed. Since four of the five compassionate reassignments were rejected due to Lyme Disease, I certainly want to know why The National Academy is not listing any studies on this infectious diseases.

Each state is responsible for providing information to their citizens. It was interesting how each of the fifty states differed regarding Lyme Disease. The cases reported in each state reflects the CDC's report for the years 1993-2001.

Alaska. The "North to The Future" state. Visiting their Department of Health (DOH) website (as I will for each and every state to see what I can learn about how they portray Lyme Disease to the residents), I found a bulletin #25, dated September 1991 that states "Alaska is one of four states that have not reported indigenous Lyme Disease". No other statistics were given and the website was difficult to navigate. Shame of you Alaska! Your citizens do travel and if they don't get Lyme Disease in your state, they may get it on a trip. They live in Alaska and should be able to find information, especially about a disease that is right up on the charts with HIV/AIDS and Cancer. Seven cases have been reported to CDC for your state (1993-2001).

Alabama, "We Dare Defend Our Rights". They have what is called the Alabama Center for Health Statistics and was last updated with any reports in 2002. I could not find Lyme Disease listed separately, but found 7,706 "all other cases" (so I am assuming that Lyme Disease is somewhere in this number), were reportable diseases (reportable to the CDC). The navigation is incredibly difficult and leaves a lot to be desired in the way of information. Citizens of Alabama, defend your right to up-to-date information and how it appears on this website. You have had 102 cases reported.

The "God Enriches" state is Arizona. God help them should anyone need to find information on their DOH website for Lyme Disease. There was nothing listed concerning this disease. This state reports 14 cases.

Arkansas, "The People Rule" state reports 114 cases. On their DOH website, CDC granted $70,000.00 to study the issues of falls and fires experienced by the elderly (2000-2001 ADA annual report). Lyme Disease was not listed under "Diseases", the site was extremely difficult to navigate and very little useful information.

California is known for the "Eureka", in layman's terms, "I have found it". There are 969 reported cases and it looks like the ticks have found your state and citizens. However, there is no information on your DOH website that would even suggest anyone in your health department knows the ticks have been dwelling there. Please find the information and post it for your residents. They are infected!

Colorado, "Nothing Without The Diety". There are 4 reported cases as listed by CDC. Remember that CDC says that Lyme Disease is at least underreported by 10%. This could actually mean you have 40 cases and only a brief fact sheet posted on your website. There is room for improvement here.

Connecticut with 24,348 cases is the number two state for reported Lyme Disease. "He who transplanted still sustains" is their state motto and I believe it. The disease is there, transplanted from somewhere and is sustaining better than the thousands who have been infected. In 2001, a reporting format was adopted in this fine state. It says that Lyme Disease is to be reported within twelve hours of recognition or suspicion, as it is for HIV and Typhoid Fever. The disease was realized in 1977 (Lyme Connecticut), but it took the CDC five years (1982) to start a surveillance. It took another five years (1987) before it became mandatory for physicians to report Lyme Disease and another year (1988) before Laboratories were required to report to CDC. The website is easily navigated and it even has a Kids' Lyme Disease site.

Delaware, with 1,150 reported cases with 189 cases between 2000-2002. The site is not fancy and only has one small paragraph about the disease. It states what some of the symptoms are and Lyme Disease is supposed to be reported within two days of lab-confirmation or clinical diagnosis. Their state motto is "Liberty and Independence". Set your citizens free with information, Delaware.

D.C., "Justice to All". I will believe that when I see it since I do not feel that any justice was forthcoming in our case. But, then maybe you have to live there to get justice. When I tried to locate their DOH, it was impossible. I can go to their homepage and pay a traffic ticket, learn about the city and even find a restaurant. But, nothing about Lyme Disease. Interesting! The capitol of our nation and the hub of information, but nothing about the disease that is stopping us from living our lives. Wake up Washington, D.C., you have 69 reported cases.

Florida, the Sunshine state and uses "In God We Trust" as their state motto. They hail with 413 cases and have actually reported study findings. Yeah, Florida! Not enough, but on the right path. I have spoken with some Florida residents and there seems to be a common theory about one of the ways the disease may be spreading. Since we know that the disease is more prevalent in the North East, and mulch is harvested from this area for distribution, could it be that the disease is spread through mulch delivered to other states? I believe there's a high possibility and this should be another study. Maybe someone can figure out how to treat the mulch before it is shipped.

Georgia, also another good website, is welcomed into the tick infested world with 200 cases of Lyme Disease. Their PDF files are not worth reading because they mimic what the CDC puts out on their site. However, I was thrilled that they say they are doing studies within the state and are educating health care providers. "Wisdom, Justice, and Moderation" is their state motto.

Hawaii has only 2 cases reported and the only state between 1993 and 2001 to have three years where the disease was classified as "not notifiable". Ua mau ke ea o ka aina i ka pono (The life (sovereignty) of the land is
perpetuated in (by) righteousness) is their motto. I searched their website and found West Nile Virus and SARS, but no mention of Lyme Disease. In their 2003 Annual Report, I found a wonderful study on student alcohol, tobacco and other drug use study, what they are planning for mental health, water and air quality and again, West Nile Virus. With two cases (which could be as many as 20 or more), it's time Hawaii at least address this on their website.

Idaho, Esto perpetua (may it endure forever) may fir the state when it comes to Lyme Disease. On the latest bulletin I could find listed (dates July 1999), Under "What About Lyme Disease in Idaho?", it stated that there were 42 cases in 1989 with an average of two cases per year. It went on to insinuate that the 42 cases could be from laboratory error and/or because these cases were reported on clinical diagnosis alone. They suggest that the CDC's recommendation of the 2-part test (ELISA and Western blot) is for confirmation. This state, between 1993 and 2001, had thirty cases reported. Clinical diagnosis or otherwise, there are Lyme Disease infected ticks in Idaho and the website needs updating immediately.

Illinois, "State sovereignty, national union" motto and comes in with 182 cases under their reporting belt. Their website is confusing. A report for 2001 states that there were no cases of Lyme Disease and CDC reports that they had 32 cases. Does this say that the Illinois Health Department isn't receiving the reports before they go to CDC? Someone in charge check the facts please. And, while you are at it, please update the website with necessary and reliable Lyme Disease information. It's behind the times and a Lymer can't afford for this to happen.

Indiana, you should be ashamed of yourself. You being the "Crossroads of America" should have something better to offer than an outdated website regarding Lyme Disease. I have spoken with Dr. Robert Pinger (Ball State University) and Dr. James Howell (Indiana University) and found that neither of you addressed the problems with Lyme Disease fully. Dr. Pinger stated that the tick collection program was out of funds for two years and Dr. Howell stated that he had 17 other more important diseases he was concentrating on. There are reports dating back to the 80's from Dr. Pinger about this disease. When I asked for information, he led me to believe that there was not much done in the way of learning about his in Indiana. I asked Dr. Howell, in October 2003, to consider updating the website (he said that he would try to get some updated information and possibly links by the end of March 2004). I polled residents from Indiana and found that most do not believe this disease is a problem here. Guess again my fine friends! It is here and there have been 244 cases reported (translates to 2,440 by CDC's criteria). Deer hunting is a big past time here and people of all ages participate. This means they are in the woods, carting the deer with the ticks home, and eating meat from infected deer, that if undercooked, could pose a serious problem. According to the tick plotting map, we are covered with infected ticks. It should not take five months to change the website with information you already have. In order to actually BE the Crossroad of America, you have to be part of the system and let your citizens that this is a real disease (you list currently that Lyme Disease may have a symptom such as arthritis), there are no treatment facilities, but links to help would be appreciated. Unless the people know from responsible agencies that it's actually in the state and what they can look for, you become part of the problem instead of part of the solution.

Iowa comes in with 189 cases and lives under the motto, "our liberties we prize and our rights we will maintain". In Iowa, one can report Lyme Disease by phone or mail, but when I looked at their "reportable disease by decade", under Lyme, there was nothing entered. Here's a wake up call, Iowa. Now is the time to concentrate on Lyme Disease along with that giant obesity study.

Kansas has a Lyme Disease information sheet on their website and 182 cases are reported according to the CDC 1993-2001 report. After reading several news flashes posted on the site, I see that West Nile Virus (WNV) is still the number one concern. There are many paragraphs covering the WNV and a warning each active mosquito season. Do they want to warn their citizens that Lyme Disease carrying ticks are ever present and can infect at any time? Hello, Lyme Disease calling Kansas! Your motto may be "as astra per aspera" (to the stars through difficulties), but you don't have to have difficulties getting the information out to your faithful residents. Be a star, instead of reaching for one.

Kentucky, the "land of tomorrow", comes to us with 184 cases of Lyme Disease. The website is nice and even includes pictures of the ticks and the bulls eye rash. You won't find Lyme Disease listed under Communicable Disease Programs (only HIV/AIDS, STDs, and TB), but under Diseases or Conditions, Lyme Disease is described. They state that it first became known in 1975 (only two years off from other sites) and that blood tests may be confusing depending on the stage of the disease (good for you, Kentucky!). However, you have one serious website problem. You state that there is a vaccine (and I am guess here, but LYMErix is probably what you are referring to), available. It was removed from the market and should be removed from your site immediately. Other than that, Kudos!

Louisiana had a reported 78 cases and a definite lacking of Lyme Disease information on their website. What I did find was their "2003 Health Report Card" (released February 2004). One line caught my eye about no health department can effectively prevent or control diseases without knowledge of when and where the cases are coming from. I found the usual, STDs, HIV/AIDS, and TB, the cost of taking care of an AIDS patient is about $85,000.00 over their lifetime, and that dog bite injuries and cancer warranted a mention, but Lyme Disease didn't pass the muster. Louisiana, an "F" on your report card. Lyme Disease is just as important as HIV/AIDS and costs more in the long run if not treated. Your state motto,
"Union, Justice, and Confidence" is one we should all live by. Union with all other states and countries to diagnose, treat and get rid of this disease; justice for all the Lyme Disease victims because it does not seem there is any for us out there; and confidence that everyone is doing their part to actively seek answers (in spite of funds, teams, or opinions).

Maine, "Dirigo" (I lead) is their motto. In with 491 cases of Lyme Disease and a website that is a rich in resources, they lead so far in my visits with each state's website. In Maine, Lyme Disease is reportable via phone, fax or mail within 48 hours. Lyme Disease is an option on the right of the screen. It took me to a serene colored background and the face of a deer. It listed symptoms, tick removal, protection, and additional links (the links could use expansion). What I was most impressed with is that there is actually a Lyme Disease contact person with the email address and phone number. Maine Medical Center Research Institute is listed at the link site and clinical trials are updated daily. There was one study (NYSPI IRB 3613) being done at the NY State Psychiatric Institute. You can also register to be notified of other clinical trials on up to twenty topics.

Maryland, please note that you are still supporting the Lyme Disease vaccine and you state that it is 80% effective in preventing the disease. This website was last updated in May of 2000. It's time for some new information. You had 4,770 cases from 1993-2001 (more like 47,700 if it was underreported by 10%). What are you waiting for? In another report, symptoms are listed and what you should do; visit your health care provider. So there are Lyme Literate doctors in Maine? Is that why most of your residents travel to New York or North Carolina for treatment. Just reporting the cases does not solve the whole problem. Having educated physicians is the key. "Fatti Maschii, Parole Femine" (Manly Deeds, Womanly Words) is their state motto.

Massachusetts, "by the sword we seek peace, but peace only under liberty" and coming in with 5,004 cases of Lyme Disease. Diagnosing Lyme Disease, the site states, is based on clinical signs and symptoms (yeah!). This sight is aggressive and informative. It recommends that physicians stop for new information where they can actually see a bulls eye rash and a suggested treatment plan. How clever is this? It would be even better is the treatment weren't limited to two weeks of antibiotics with a repeat if symptoms persist. But, the site does list co-infections and treatments. Why would I expect anyone to be on the same sheet of music since patients differ, the symptoms migrate, and the standard treatment does not take all of this into play. I still have to give a thumbs up for this website.

Michigan with only 188 cases seems to be on a good path. Last report, dated Spring 2001 "Lyme Disease Testing Reminder", they state that the following tests are done free of charge at the Michigan Department of Community Health: the two-step CDC standard testing, skin biopsy of the rash, and tick identification. In this same report, I found that the CDC funded, upon recommendation by the General Accounting Office (Emerging Diseases report 1999), a project for a National Laboratory System (NLS). It looks like it is a two year project and will include assurance of complete and rapid infectious disease reporting; expedient testing; and will develop a forum for communication between labs and other public health groups. Wow! If they can actually get the medical professionals to comply with reporting, testing straightened out, and any form of communication done in two years, I believe I would eat a tick. CDC cannot find a way to test accurately for this disease. The cases of Lyme Disease are underreported by at least 10% and this is since 1982. And communication? No one can positively say that one treatment is better than another because every case is different as the patients are different. When a doctor tries to treat the patient with what is working for that individual, some government agency comes along and wants to control that treatment (OMPC in New York is prime example of headhunting doctors). So, if Michigan can actually get even one of these tasks in place, it is much more than is being accomplished in this area to date. I suspect that this new NLS is mainly for bioterrorism, however. That's just the impression I got from the report. Their motto is "if you seek a pleasant peninsula, look about you."

Minnesota, the "star oh the north", has a reported 2,534 cases of Lyme Disease up through 2001. Although the website is chuck full of information, a couple of things stood out for me. It was stated that there was no current evidence that suggested a patient who tested positive with symptoms of Lyme Disease should receive antibiotics. Excuse me? We go because of symptoms, are clinically diagnosed with Lyme Disease and follow up with the required testing. It comes back positive (but they say that there are false positives and negatives) and we still should not be able to receive medication because the symptoms have subsided or migrated? This site lists Mayo Clinic as a resource. When I went to the Mayo Clinic site for treatment, it stated that antibiotics are recommended for early stages of Lyme Disease and hospitalization and/or IV drug therapy for later stages. So, if you have early stage Lyme Disease, seek treatment, the tests come back positive, but some of the symptoms have eased or migrated, antibiotics are not recommended? I would again like to suggest that every state get on the same sheet of music here. It's not a totally different disease folks. It's Lyme Disease that may have (and hopefully are tested for) co-infections. It's no wonder Lyme Disease victims cannot get treated. They also state that the testing may be confusing because there is no standardized testing (reasons for false positive/negatives), the protocols for treatment are different from state to state, and there isn't enough education or clinical studies.

By this time, I am almost discouraged. I am starting to see what Lymers from across the country are raising so much hell about. I hear that testing at different labs is not good and their doctors don't truly believe they have Lyme Disease and most are unwilling to treat it, etc. This could be a whole lot less frustrating if everyone recognized the need for unification. Then, maybe the insurance companies and drug companies would have to join the party.

Mississippi does not have an impressive site in regards to Lyme Disease. It has a fact sheet, but with 100 reported cases, one would think that there would be more. I wasn't expecting positive answers to is it sexually transmitted or is there a cure. The site just left me wanting more than a page with almost the same wording as the CDC site. The one good idea they have implemented is recruiting doctors from around the nation to work in under-served areas. We can only hope that these physicians are educated in the area of clinically diagnosing Lyme Disease. State motto is "by valor and arms".

United we stand, divided we fall rings as Missouri's state motto. With 511 cases reported and a really nice motto, I was hoping to find Lyme Disease information that would put the other sites to shame (not that most of them could bear much more humiliation). Missouri is know as the "show me" state. I would like them to considering showing me where, if there are any, reports about this disease is on their website. I found a couple publications that could be ordered, but nothing for the Lyme Disease patient to reference. And to top it off, the site was hard to get around and not pleasing to the eye. Get busy Missouri. Looks like you have a lot of catching up to do.

Montana (who reports no cases of Lyme Disease and deny

that they have ticks that carry this disease) was selected (as was Michigan and 15 other sites) to participate in the three year program (I believe Michigan said it was two years, but this could be just another reporting error or not the same study at all) that will develop a tracking system for infectious diseases. This program is 100% federally funded and each year, the site will receive $510,000.00 to support the study. This is the only information that I was able to recover from Montana at this time. The state motto is "gold and silver".

Nebraska, "equality before the law" is how they claim to live. With only 46 cases of Lyme Disease up through 2001, maybe there are only a few criminal ticks residing in this fine state. But, one villain is one too many. And their site, being very difficult to find Lyme Disease tucked away, I did find that Nebraska claims that they have no solid evidence that anyone has contracted Lyme Disease in their state, even with cases being reported to CDC for Nebraska. I even double checked, and sure enough, there were 46 cases by 2001. The very least they could do on the site is offer their residents links since someone may actually believe they didn't get the disease there and therefore, cannot be treated in Nebraska.

Nevada has buried Lyme Disease so far into the area that it was difficult to locate. I know that 32 cases may not seem like many to some people, but even one case is worth the effort to post up-to-date information and offer even that one victim a place to turn. They probably feel all alone with this disease anyway, why would any state run website alienate them further? Your motto, "all for our country" says it all...give your all, including Lyme Disease information on your website.

New Hampshire, the "live free, or die" state hails with 444 Lyme Disease cases. Well, I hate to say this, but after browsing the Health Department's website, I could not find Lyme Disease listed. I did find SARS and HIV, but that was not surprising. Seems that in this state, you won't find a whole lot of assistance posted on the website.

New Jersey has a fairly good website and it's easy to get around on it. Information about Lyme Disease was readily available, but nothing interesting. However, the links are worth the trip. One a scale of 1-10, with 10 being the highest score, I would have to give New Jersey a 7. With "Liberty and Prosperity" being the state's motto and 16,362 of Lyme Disease up through 2001, I wish their citizens my best in locating treatment.

New Mexico, "it grows as it goes" and known as the land of enchantment with only 16 reported cases of Lyme Disease, I had hoped to be able to locate a reasonably informative site. But, alas, when I looked at all the reports available and then did a word search ("Lyme Disease"), nothing came up. No mention of it. This is an embarrassment and I hope that before any grants are given to New Mexico for any health care studies, they are compelled to add one of the most emerging diseases since HIV/AIDS.

New York, the leader in Lyme Disease cases (38,538 through 2001) and "excelsior" (fine curled wood shavings used especially for packing fragile items, according to the Merriam-Webster online dictionary) as their state motto, I was actually surprised to find very little useful information on their website. With that many Lyme Disease victims, I would have surmised that this would be the website to go to for information. However, there is nothing there worth reading about the disease. One would be better off going to an on-line support group for information. This is disgraceful and an injustice to a group of citizens that have already been through the torrid of hell. With as many fine doctors in New York willing and able to treat this disease, they should be listed in bold script under the Lyme Disease heading.

North Carolina, "to be rather than to seem" is the state's motto and an overstatement. When does the co-infections of Lyme Disease warrant more space than the disease itself? The one small paragraph had very little information and not worth visiting. With 572 cases, it would be a gesture of concern if residents could go to the one place in their state that they look to for information and updates. Lyme Disease is real and spreading like fire. The day is today and the time is now to get the information right and posted for victims to start getting assistance where they live...not where they have to travel to.

North Dakota, " liberty and union, now and forever, one and inseparable" and sever cases of Lyme Disease under their oneness. However, don't bother to search for Lyme Disease on their website because it isn't there. SARS and HIV are listed, as well as influenza, but somehow, North Dakota missed the top ten list of infectious diseases. Get with it North Dakota!

Ohio had 82 cases of Lyme Disease in 2002 (376 cases from 1993-2001). Their website had less than the basics regarding Lyme Disease. I hope that their state motto, "with God all things are possible", will be able to get their residents through this disease. I believe in God and pray that each day will be better than the one before. So far, I am still suffering with Lyme Disease, living in purgatory because of the way the military deals with this disease, and still begging each state to get on board. I will pray for you Ohio.

Oklahoma, the state where I personally got this disease, was hard for me to write about. It may have been seven years ago and I can barely remember life before Lyme Disease, but I hold the military installation and the state's Department of Health responsible for not making the information readily available. "Labor conquers all things"? Well, that's their motto and from where I sit, if they labored any less where Lyme Disease is concerned, they wouldn't have the few unimportant reports they have on the website. There were 290 Lyme Disease cases between 1993-2001. In fact, Oklahoma states on their reports that 1991 was the first year that Lyme Disease was reportable by law. I was totally under the assumption that CDC started making this reportable since 1982 (when they first started collecting information on this disease). On their "Table of Selected Reportable Diseases" dated January 1-December 31, 2003, Lyme Disease wasn't even on the list. When I was diagnosed at Ft. Sill, Oklahoma, I am thrilled that I didn't go to the Oklahoma Department of Health website for information. I would have given up then because I would have been lead to believe that there was no information and therefore, no hope. However, those that live on hope will soon die from starvation. So, unless you want to offer your residents only hope to survive on, I would suggest the website be updated with current information. And there's no time like the present.

Oregon is not one of the best websites for Lyme Disease information. It relies on CDC links to explain the disease for them. Their motto is "she flies with her own wings" and angels need to get into the website and update the information. With 137 cases, it would be fair for me to say that there are more than 1,370 patients who could use updated information and direction to anyone there that could help them receive treatment. Let's not rely solely on CDC.

Pennsylvania "Virtue, Liberty, and Independence" reports in with 19,777 cases of Lyme Disease. Their web site lists Ehrlichiosis, but to find Lyme Disease, you have to go to "about us", click on this and that and this again....so buried. There is a good reason they hid their take on Lyme Disease, it's out dated and no links to better information. I would think that with the possibility of 197,770 cases, I would be able to locate pertinent Lyme Disease information. Shape up Pennsylvania.

Rhode Island, shame on you! The website is not even noteworthy when talking about Lyme Disease. And your state reports 5,484 cases from 1993-2001 and another 852 in 2002, alone. Translated into real numbers, looks like about 63,360 or more cases. And you couldn't find information or links to post that would direct your citizens to treatment? Remember that some Lymers have lost cognitive skills and things need to be plain and simple for us. But, there actually has to be something there to begin with and your site is lacking. "Hope" is your state motto. I just "hope" that you will update your website and get with the program. Your citizens deserve no less.

South Carolina, the "prepared in mind and resources" state. Their website, as many others leave a lot to be desired. I did learn that between 1993-2001, there were 6 reported cases of Lyme Disease and 26 cases in 2002. For this kind of increase, I would expect to find better information. It's time to get the minds of your state together and figure out what resources you can offer your residents that suffer with Lyme Disease.

South Dakota, "under God the people rule", and with only 1 reported case between 1993-2001. The web site, compared to the number of cases, is actually well done. There's not a wealth of information, but there is enough to get anyone with Lyme Disease started on their path to answers.

Tennessee is another sad site for Lyme Disease information. If you believe the written report, it looks like there were 22 cases in 2002. If you read the file report, it appears to be 24 cases. All in all, the cases reported to CDC between 1993-2001 was 295. And no information on the site that is useful. "Agriculture and commerce" is the state motto. Isn't there communication used for agriculture and commerce? There are at least 3,190 residents of Tennessee that would appreciate your concern with their disease.

Texas, the "friendship" state. Their website is friendly and Lyme Disease is out there for the residents to find. I lived in Texas for over a year and found that the doctors who were Lyme literate were more common in the northern and eastern side of the state. The last update to the website was reported to be in December 2003. Here, it states that the disease was uncovered in 1976 (we have reports that range from 1975-1978) and was only found in Texas in 1984. In 2002, there were 133 cases and 594 cases between 1993-2001. I believe that Texas would be a good place for treatment, but TriCare would not allow me to see any of their educated doctors.

Utah is known for their "industry" motto. Their website is mediocre, but has the basic information and a couple of links for more information. There were 14 reported cases in the state between 1993-2001.

Vermont, "freedom and unity", the website has basic information with the exception of treatment. The only link on the Lyme fact sheet is to the CDC. There were 166 reported cases.

Virginia, "mountaineers are always free", and your website is very nice and informative. There were 905 cases reported through 2001 and it looks like you have taken this disease seriously. It reflects in how you have your website set up and the amount of information you provide for your residents. My hat off to you!

Washington, "Alki" is a Chinook Indian term they use for their state motto. It means "bye-bye" or "hope for the future". This site is the best of the best. There are pages and pages of Lyme Disease information and even goes as far to state that clinical diagnosis is recommended with blood tests to support (not diagnose). This is the site if you want in depth information in a clear concise format. If there were awards (and I believe this is a good idea), Washington State would be the winner, hands down. With 91 cases reported through 2001, they go the extra mile for their Lyme Disease residents and much further in educating their physicians (if they use the website) than most states.

West Virginia has a brown background website Lyme Disease Fact Sheet. No new stuff here and pretty much what you would find on any "do the least we can do" website. They reported 211 cases through 2001 and seem to share the same state motto with Virginia.

Wisconsin, "forward", and another simple basic information fact sheet. With 4,430 cases, I was expecting bigger and better.

Wyoming, the "equal rights" state, with 32 cases of Lyme Disease and a sight that can almost be said to have no information. When I searched the site for Lyme Disease, it returned one report that mentioned the disease. In the article, Lyme Disease came up because they wanted to point out how someone could get the disease, being outdoors. It's time to give equal rights to Lyme Disease.

So, many states mention the basics, some don't bother and so few make the information readily available. Even state to state, I can see that it will be a long time before everyone is making the effort to post accurate information designed to educate, direct and support the victims of Lyme Disease.

There are other countries who have concerns with this disease. I approached doctors from other countries and of all the emails I sent out, very few replied. From the few responses I received, I would be safe in assuming that they did not reply because there were no studies being conducted or trials they could talk about. From Dusseldorf Germany, Dr. Hemmer was not aware of any study in Germany; Dr. Klempner in the U.S.A. said that I should go to the NIAID website for any currently funded studies lists; Dr. Phillip Baker, NIH was very helpful and instructed me where to find clinical trials listed on their website; John Halperin with the Naval Medical Education and Training Command, USA let me know that I should contact two doctors in Boston to ask about any studies they may be doing; Volker Fingerle from Germany said that he had no information about clinical trials in the near future; Thomas Kamradt, Germany referred me to NIH; and Dr. Juan Carlos Garcia-Monco, Department of Neurology, Hospital de Galdacano, Vizcaya, Spain was not aware of any clinical trials at the present time.

Where do we go from here? Do I dare to believe that the pharmaceutical or insurance companies are doing anything to provide better medications, testing or coverage?

CHAPTER X

The Internet and Answers

Coming back to the Midwest was a traumatic experience in itself, but having Lyme Disease and now being dirt poor left me totally depressed. The first three months, I could not grasp the depths of despair and could see no light at the end of the tunnel.

Tim was now working long hours again, but at least he was within a phone call should I need him. Many times, I did. I was confused more and more, the pain seemed to be increasing and I wasn't sleeping well again. We were living off handouts and cheap hot dogs. And no matter how many letters I wrote to the Army, we were no closer to getting this straightened out than when it had all begun.

I contacted Sheila (not her real name) who had assisted me with support at the start of this humiliating plea for help. She was busy with saving doctors in New York. She said that there were headhunters looking to take out doctors that treated Lyme Disease there. I could hardly believe my ears! How could anyone deny a physician from treating a disease? I would later learn that if the good guys treated this disease, but didn't follow the "Steere" guidelines, they were prosecuted. Not only were the guidelines not reasonable because they didn't take into account that each patient was different, but they didn't make sense because there were so many strains and reports from many physicians stated that some were resistant to antibiotic therapy. If the patient was getting better or maintaining, wasn't this cause to keep up the treatment? From what I was understanding, if I had been given longer antibiotic treatment in the beginning, I may have not ended up to be a Chronic Lymer (the reason that the Army would not approve a compassionate reassignment). If I were not a chronic Lyme Disease victim, then there would have been no reason to ask for a compassionate reassignment. And, if we wouldn't have needed a compassionate reassignment, then Tim would not be AWOL for trying to save my life. But, what is done is done and we can never go back.

Even though Sheila was extremely busy, offered to find someone to help me get my story out and try to clear this mess up. She thought that going to the media would be a good thing and make the whole country aware that an active duty soldier was being denied the right to care for his very ill wife.

Paula called me the very next day. She was another Lymer, but her specialty had been publicity before she became bedridden with this disease. Paula was a wonderful woman and revealed her story to me. It was heart wrenching. To have a whole life of good things and then to have everything taken away by a tick. She and her husband were white collar professionals with two teenage children. They had what I call the "American home lifestyle". She became ill, her husband nearly lost his business and they were struggling. Hey! wait a minute, this sounds like my story. They weren't eating hot dogs or having to beg to borrow $20.00 until pay day, but they were struggling just the same.

Paula quietly listened to my story. I told her my life from the day I was diagnosed right through to the point we were at. This was only the second time I had ever cried since the military had listed Tim as AWOL. Even when we had to share a meal, I felt closer to my husband. When we had to dumpster-dive for things, I looked at it as a new experience. When we sold my grandmother's last few trinkets or pawned my wedding rings, I never shed a tear. Tim and I lived by "improvise, adapt, and overcome" when it came to life in the military. But, telling Paula the story brought so many emotions to the surface that I could not contain the tears. Paula said that she would be happy to assist me in making media contacts.

Paula and I worked on a press release until it said it all.

Army Classifies Soldier Deserter as he tries to save his Wife.

Always putting his duty to the Armed Forces of the United States and his country first, Staff Sergeant Tim Vogan served the Army for over 19 years with a spotless record. During his eighth month in Korea of his last tour, his extremely active wife, Sue Vogan became seriously ill. Tim requested a mid tour leave to assist his wife with her medical care and was granted one. While on leave, by his wife's side, Sue suffered a heart attack, underwent surgery, and developed serious lung problems. Staff Sergeant Vogan immediately asked for a compassionate reassignment because Sue had no one but him to help care for her and her physicians were insisting on Tim's presence. He was refused 4 times. Sue also suffers from co-infections from Lyme disease, a degenerative spine, her cognitive skills have been severely impaired by Lyme, her eyesight is failing, and is presently on oxygen. Denying this Veteran Noncommissioned Officer a compassionate reassignment while his wife became critical was shocking, but when his pay and all benefits ceased in March, the Vogans were outraged. Staff Sergeant Vogan is only 3 months away from retirement and now with no money and no benefits, Sue has been without medicine for 2 months.

Being a good soldier, Tim Vogan sent another desperate letter to his command, but no reply came. Now he is classified as AWOL and faces many penalties, after a life time of excellent service to the Army. The Vogans finally contacted Congressman Michael Oxley of Ohio, and Congressman Christopher Smith of New Jersey to help them with a Congressional investigation as to why the Surgeon General of the Army, who has had Staff Sergeant Vogan's requests for 3 months, will not address the reassignment and the AWOL classification.

Sue also gave her life to the Army while holding down two jobs at times. She helped new families in service, raised money, volunteered for Red Cross, NCO Wives, Army Community Services, American Cancer Society, Ft. Sill Commissary Focus Group, Ft. Sill's International Student Division, Family Support Group Leader, called by other commands for assistance, was an instructor and lead fundraiser for Army Family Team Building, adopted 54 South Korean orphans, and just before she became ill, sent out over 300 boxes to servicemen in Iraq. Sue also helped the local civilian community. She was in charge of decorating the downtown area for Christmas, assisted a local foster care program, opened their home at Thanksgiving and Christmas for stay-back soldiers giving them a traditional meal, gifts, and a free call home to their loved ones, substituting for a local school, served two chair positions at a local civilian hospital, and assisted with abused military wives. Now that the Vogans desperately need the Army, the Army has deserted them.

Paula sent this out to her list of media contacts and within a couple of days, I received a call from a producer at CBS. He was so understanding and wanted an exclusive with us. Finally, the story would break and the military would have to admit that they made a mistake, but would clear it all up. We would actually be able to pay our bills again and get my treatment for this awful disease.

Tim called the attorney we had in mind to take our case should we ever find $15,000.00 while dumpster-diving. The advice was for Tim not to appear on television or say a word. I just didn't understand this. When an injustice has been done, intentionally or by mistake, the parties involved should have the right to straighten it out. We didn't like the idea of airing this, but we were at the end of our rope. We followed the chain of command as we had been taught to do, respected the advice from the Pentagon down to the lowest command, but we were no better off than the day I received the letter stating that Tim was AWOL. Tim again followed advice and CBS cancelled the interview. Now, no one would ever know. The military's secret was safe and we would be forever sentenced to this place. My world, as hellish as it had become, finally came crashing down and I sunk into a deep depression.

There we were, no hope and only each other to rely on again. Most days, we didn't even discuss the issues or make any plans. How could we, Tim was listed as AWOL and I had chronic Lyme Disease? We weren't really part of the civilian world and the military had forsaken us. We were not in heaven and we weren't in hell. It was the in-between area that some call purgatory. We just knew it was numbing and depressing.

After all of the hard work and my researching this disease, I could not find one glimmer of light. There were no doctors in the military that treated Lyme Disease. There were no doctors here that treated Lyme Disease. And, from what I heard from New York, this disease would never be treated because all the good doctors would soon be out of practice.

TriCare was no help, but then we didn't have them anymore. The new insurance was another HMO and seemed to be as bad as TriCare. They wanted you to have a PCP and expected this physician to treat it all. I expected that this was their way to save them money and they could control my healthcare. Where were we supposed to go from here?

I went to the online support groups. There, I didn't feel so alone. When someone mentioned that they were having pain or sleepless nights, I could actually relate. Not like when someone outside the Lyme circle states that they had a rough night sleeping. Very different.

My mother was empathetic when I told her that I had Lyme Disease. She went so far as to get a little information on this disease. However, she didn't understand. She offered her home remedies and suggested what worked for her when she had a pain. When I visited her, she told me that I looked fine. The symptoms aren't displayed on our faces, so people think we are fine or that we are faking.

Now, I ask you, why in the hell would anyone want to fake this disease? Why would a person want to be on unpleasant extended therapy or give up their sex life just to save their spouse from getting it? Why in God's name would anyone enjoy secluding themselves because they stutter and can't find words to express themselves? This disease is real and needs validation. I was always proud of being healthy. I loved life and all the activity thrown my way. I have always hated sympathy expressed for me, even before this disease. Now that I am ill, I like sympathy even less, if that's possible. Lyme Disease is sucking all the life out of my days.

The more that people told me I looked fine, the more I stayed away from people. The computer became my best friend and it could take me to places I never imagined.

After searching for help through many contacts made with

the pharmaceutical companies, I gave up. These people kept referring me back to NIH or CDC. When I asked CDC what was being
done, I received a very vague reply by email. They responded by
telling me that they work with NIH and FDA, among other agencies. And, if I wanted any more information, it was suggested that I
contact NIH. When I contacted NIH, I was told that they had a list
of studies (3 at present) and was free to contact them to enroll.
However, hardly anyone I know qualifies for these studies. I
learned that NIH set the criteria for the studies, but it looked like
they were way off base. The studies didn't seem to be geared to actually finding the treatment for this disease. I was disappointed.

Profits and low overhead seemed to be what insurance companies were all about. The few doctors that were said to be treating
Lyme Disease were being hunted up like wild dogs. The pharmaceutical companies were not working on any studies. Why aren't we
being helped? Why wasn't this illness being addressed or more relief offered?

I recalled the history of this disease and went back to the beginning and Dr. Allen Steere seemed to be the starting point. I
pulled up all of the abstracts and articles that I could possibly find
that included his name. I wanted to know why there was no help,
no new information and very few doctors who treated this disease.
There had to be answers if I went to the beginning and came forward. The following is my timeline according to Dr. Steere's abstracts:

1978-April; Symptomatic treatment only is advised, except in
the rare instances of severe neurologic complications or myocardial
conduction abnormality.

1979- June; Chronic Lyme arthritis resembles RA pathologi-
cally, but differs in two important ways.

1980- July; Clinical manifestations of the disease may fluc-
tuate from year to year and influence apparent antibiotic effect --
twenty patients were studied who had cardiac problems with Lyme
Disease and the clinical picture included that complete heart blockage may be commoner.

1983- July; Out of 108 patients studied, nearly half of the patients had major late symptoms that were as they were before
treatment.

1984- July; Weeks to months later, some patients develop

neurologic or cardiac problems, intermittent attacks of arthritis which may become chronic with erosion of cartilage and bone -- facial palsies, motor and sensory problems and weakness.

1985- February; recognition of the clinical picture remains very important in diagnosing early Lyme Disease.

1986- December; Evidence suggests that Lyme Disease occurs in stages with different clinical manifestations at each stage, but the course of the illness in each patient is highly variable.

1987- February; All 3 stages of Lyme Disease can be treated with antibiotic therapy, but some patients with late disease may not respond.

1988- ...immunologic damage in response to persistence of the spirochete, however few number.

1989- August; Treatment with appropriate antibiotics is usually curative, but longer courses of therapy are often needed later in the illness, and some patients may not respond.

1990-November; Chronic neurologic manifestations of Lyme Disease suggests that antibiotic is necessary

1999- Protests against Dr. Steere for being honored as "astute clinician" at NIH - it is stated that Dr. Steere brought his "overdiagnosis and overtreatment" school of thought to the forefront and thereby has put physicians, that treat Lyme Disease aggressively, into danger of losing their careers. He is also cited for being the reason we are now turned away for treatment.

What happened to Dr. Steere, father of Lyme Disease? He seemed to be heading in the right direction, from diagnosing the disease to finding that it had three stages. And only ten years ago, he saw that longer treatment was necessary and that some of us would not respond to the therapy. Is it because research money was being directed to Steere followers, as rumors suggested? Was this shift in position due to political pressure? Why would anyone, without clinical proof, set up guidelines that do not allow full treatment for a patient? Does this happen with cancer patients? Are they only entitled to X amount of days on treatment? Is the AIDS community being subjected to standards that make it almost impossible to get well?

I noticed that the CDC page has referenced Dr. Steere many times. Is this the reason that CDC still uses outdated criteria? Is Dr. Steere the reason that newer testing is not used?

I worked for a laboratory and we were involved with Gulf War Illness a few years ago. I recalled that Professor Garth Nicolson was doing wonders with testing, so I decided to contact him. If there was one intelligent and honorable man, it was Professor Nicolson.

It would turn out that not only was the Professor gracious, but had already developed tests that is more sensitive and accurate in regards to Lyme Disease.

"We have completed our study of Borrelia-positive Lyme pts. The majority (>65%) have mycoplasmal infections, mostly Mycoplasma fermentans (similar to the Gulf War veterans but unlike most civilians CFS pts with mycoplasmal infections who have a variety of mycoplasmal species, including M. pneumoniae, M. hominis, M. penetrans AND M. fermentans). MDL Labs in Mt. Laurel, NJ have found very similar results with LD pts. Interestingly, in North America the most common mycoplasma specie in CFS pts is M. pneumoniae but in Europe it is M. hominis. Most pts also have multiple infections in N. America but not in Europe. In contrast in mycoplasma-positive GWI pts (40% of all GWI pts) almost all have either M. fermentans (>80%) or M. genitalium (>10%), which is rally quite unlike the civilian CFS pts (with the exception of the prison guards in selected Texas prisons where M. fermentans was being tested before the Gulf War).

Prof. Garth Nicolson

That information is on our website, www.immed.org. Look under clinical testing (also suggested Borrelia testing for CFS pts). Information is also posted under Infectious Disease Research, Gulf War Illness Research and Fatiguing Illnesses Research."

When I investigated further, I learned that this peer reviewed testing was presented to the government, but they decline to recognize it. I cannot imagine why. This information is valuable and could save thousands of dollars in testing and retesting. It would actually do some good for those of us suffering from this dreadful disease.

Does the government not want us to get well or are they afraid that we will learn where the disease came from? When there is something this accurate available, why isn't it being spread far and wide? I suppose the answer lies in the word "government". After the refusal of a compassionate reassignment for a life and death situation, I can only imagine why the tests are being ignored.

I still was left with more questions. Who put Dr. Steere in charge of guidelines and why? Weren't there other clinicians studying Lyme Disease and found that treatments, for some, needed to be extended as Dr. Steere suggested in 1989? With very few studies going on, when could we look forward to a breakthrough?

My internet support group had no answers, but I was sure thankful that they were in my life. At least I knew I was not the only one looking for a way to get back on the path to normalcy. When people say that I look fine, I would sure like to actually feel fine.

Since I could locate no other military spouse with Lyme Disease, I fell back into the civilian world. I met four wonderful souls, victims of Lyme Disease, on the internet. We formed a tight bond and spoke many times about our individual situations. Soon, we started calling each other and lending support by listening to a voice pleading to be heard. Since no one in the medical world or the government organizations would listen, we relied on each other to hear us.

In the next five chapters, you will hear from Terri, Jennifer, Carol, Ryan's mother, and my husband, Tim. They have graciously agreed to open up to you, in hopes that you may get a clearer picture of where we all are with this disease. Each deals with Lyme Disease from a different perspective. Different lifestyles and family difficulties even without Lyme Disease is never easy. But you will see the strength and courage these individuals have and one common thread...the will to live.

Chapter XI

The Disease of a Thousand Deaths

Terri's Story

Contracting neurological Lyme Disease was much easier than securing a diagnosis. In fact it was so easy, I didn't know, nor did anyone else, that I had it for thirteen years before it was discovered as the source of so many of my problems, both physical and emotional.

I must preface this story with a note that it is not easy for me to tell these things. It is very difficult to revisit the depths that this disease took me and the impact it had on my life and family. I tell it only because people need to know what symptoms Neuro Borreliosis can bring about and that recovery is possible.

In the early 1980's I was finishing graduate work on my Master of Fine Art degree in eastern North Carolina. I began having problems with my vision and my jaw hurt constantly. I lost hearing temporarily in one ear. I gained 15 pounds overnight. I took daily naps and would awaken from them unable to move and also had auditory hallucinations. I was so tired that it did not occur to me that something was wrong. Panic attacks were beginning to control my life. The jaw pain was unbearable and I eventually went to a dentist, oral surgeon, chiropractor and then an MD who sent me on to a neurologist who conducted every test he could think of. I passed but one, the visual contrast test. The doctor told me he knew that something was wrong but he did not know what. He was very kind, and told me if things got worse to let him know. I wonder where he is now?

The panic attacks and depression grew unbearable and forced me into therapy. I continued with graduate school and worked at various jobs while finishing my thesis work. I remained physically as active as I could, continuing hiking, camping, riding horses, swimming, running and gardening. I had always been comfortable outdoors. All I knew about ticks is that I didn't like them but they sure liked me.

I lived with and tried to ignore the physical pain and continued therapy for the emotional problems, obtained my graduate degree and went on to obtain a teaching certificate. After one year teaching in North Carolina I was hired to teach for the Defense Department schools and

moved to Germany. While I was there I had continued and worsened physical and emotional problems which I imagined were stress related. I had constant bronchitis or pneumonia, frequent headaches and bouts of depression. I got married and had four miscarriages. By my fourth year there, depression and panic once again took over my life. I was hospitalized after a nearly successful suicide attempt. I lay in a coma for three days. I recovered fully, but was unable to return to work. My health, both emotional and physical, spiraled downwards. I was continually ill, and by the time I left Germany, having resigned my position, I could barely make a phone call or carry out any actions that required thinking. My stress tolerance was zero and I had reached it.

I had quit drinking years before and was in fairly good physical shape but never the less I was often sick. I felt like I had the flu constantly and feared I was going crazy. Panic attacks once again ruled my life, and my familiar life-long ability to cope and my resiliency to stress were non-existent. I had bottomed out but did not know why. Neither did any doctors I saw. I was treated for depression and panic attacks along with PTSD.

Upon returning to the US, I had a complete physical. I had pneumonia. While my husband was job hunting, I was dealing with a fifth pregnancy and on the brink of another miscarriage. I found a doctor who was able to help who also urged me to apply for disability. I didn't know what that was but did as he suggested. I was soon on permanent disability, which was devastating to me. I broke down when I got my approval letter. Now I know it is part of what has saved my life. My plan was, after delivering my daughter, to give her away and then kill myself. I had chosen a friend who agreed to take her, but she talked me into sticking around. We spoke frequently. I also stayed in therapy, and as my pregnancy progressed, I began to feel a bit better. By the time my daughter was born I was happy to welcome her into the world and was thrilled to be a mom.

A few minutes after her arrival into the world, five doctors surrounded my hospital bed. They wanted orders signed for a spinal tap for her. Something was wrong. She looked perfectly normal, very healthy in fact, but she had a severe infection. They suspected but did not find meningitis. The doctors could find no bacteria in her spinal fluid but she was put on heavy doses of antibiotics for two weeks. I had to bring her every few days for a check up. No one suspected Lyme Disease, including myself.

What I knew about tick -borne disease was limited to experiences with a friend who had contracted Rocky Mountain Spotted Fever, but he had an easy diagnosis and treatment.

Divorce followed the year after the birth of my daughter and I moved from the Gulf Coast of Florida to Cape Cod. Over the course of the next few years, I continued to worsen. I had so many symptoms, fatigue so bad that I thought I surely had cancer. My mind would not

function at times and I could not do simple mental tasks. I would forget most things. I had bouts of narcolepsy. I forgot names and faces, and familiar places. My panic worsened as I would suddenly not know where I was and would become completely disoriented. My balance at times was so bad that I began to fall down. Concentration was limited to a few minutes at a time. Making a phone call was nearly impossible. I had to write down the number and cross off each one as I dialed it. I would forget who I was calling and what it was about unless I had that noted also. I forgot my daughter's name at times, and our birthdays. I dropped so many things on my feet that they were constantly black and blue.

I also forgot names of people that I knew well, and after a while I forgot their faces too. I began to withdraw socially as it was so embarrassing and very taxing to try to remember people. I was also becoming very intolerant to noises, lights and other types of sensory stimuli. Shopping was draining or impossible and I began to have someone shop for me, whenever possible.

It wasn't until later, as treatment began, that I would remember dropping something and connect that with the presence of a bruise on my foot. Many times I would search for an item, know that it was on the counter in front of me but I was unable to see it. My daughter often came to the rescue, and I made it into a game. "Mommy wants to know where the scissors are. Can you find them?" and she could. They were right in front of me.

One night while fixing dinner, I took a hot pan out of the oven with my bare hand, having forgotten to use a potholder. My daughter came toddling in the kitchen and I told her not to touch the pan, that it was hot. I moved the pan a second time to the back of the stove, and realized I had a third degree burn. I did not feel it. I knew something was terribly wrong. Pain should be a signal that something is wrong, but there wasn't any. Just blisters and redness.

I had many physical symptoms that seemed unrelated and changed constantly. My knees hurt, my feet were so painful at times I would scream, although upon examination nothing was found wrong with them. I was in and out of the ER for tremendous headaches. My neck hurt constantly and I felt like someone had screwed a metal covering onto my skull and was slowly tightening it. These would go on for days and worsen with each one. There wasn't much in the way of pain relief.

I would also have days where I felt ok, and would get the shopping done, go to the beach or ride horses. Physical exercise left me completely exhausted, yet sleep usually escaped me at night. I also began jumping out of my skin at the slightest scare or noise. I had to adjust the buzzer at my apartment as the sudden noise would cause me to fall out of my chair or drop to the floor. My ribs hurt so badly at times I could not touch them. My balance was non-existent and I broke more than one toe running into the walls. Taking a shower got to be dangerous.

All this time I was putting most of my energy into taking care of my daughter and trying to earn extra money. I did free lance art work and portraits. I arranged things in the kitchen so my daughter would be safe. I bought foods that she could get and eat herself. During times of what I called "coma sleep" I would be aware of her entering my bedroom, yet could not manage to move. I would come to every few hours and make a meal or give her a bath. I was too sick to know how sick I was. My daughter would bring her toys and books to my bed, and in between sleeping we would play games and read. She has always been independent, a quality for which I am very grateful.   Looking back on this, I am stunned that we got through this time safely. It also grieves me that we lost precious time together.

I told my doctor all of what I could remember as things happened. As I got worse, we began the process of testing and specialists and finding a diagnosis. I went through all the usual testing, MRIs, blood tests, including five Lyme titers which were negative. My doctor decided that I had sinus disease. I had surgery. It took over a year to recover from that, and my symptoms got worse. Then I was told I had CFIDS, Chronic Fatigue Immune Dysfunction Syndrome. My sinuses will still a problem so I began taking Biaxen, and I stayed on it for 8 months. It helped my other symptoms as well. When I came off that I had hallucinations and return of other symptoms within days. My doctor suspected Lyme at this point, although I had already had five negative Lyme titers. One month to the day after my last titer, I was given a Western Blot which showed I had 11 positive markers for Lyme. This was in 1996.

Treatment began. My Lyme doctor told me that I would have a Herxheimer reaction and that I would feel like I had shingles. I knew that was bad as I had known elderly people with shingles, and they were in agony. Somewhere in the midst of the following three weeks, I remembered that. I could not get out of bed without coffee and a painkiller. I had to remind myself that this painful reaction to the antibiotics was a good thing, it meant they were working.

After a few months of treatment, I began to feel better, although still a long way from well. I realized my daughter was complaining of the same type of symptoms, and had her tested as well. She was positive. So we both had Lyme. Treatment began for her in 1997.

About 8 months into treatment my Infectious Disease doctor changed the medication to tetracycline. I began to get worse. When I complained of this, he continued to tell me just to keep taking it. I spiraled downward pretty fast, and checked myself into a clinic twice. Suicidal thoughts were constant, yet I felt I could get better with correct treatment. I knew that there were other doctors available, but I did not have the resources to travel to an out of state doctor. I was not able to drive. My daughter was seeing a Lyme Pediatrician and was getting better. About two years into her treatment, I knew that if I didn't get help I would die. I returned to the Infectious Disease doctor but again was given tetracycline. I didn't bother to fill the prescription, and was told that I would not die. " No one dies from Lyme, and no one dies from AIDS" I was told. So why did I feel I was knocking on death's door?

I learned the hard way that co-infections were a large part of what was making me so sick, and I had to find a doctor that would not only treat Lyme, but address properly the other infections. That was a long hard road, and many doctors tried to help. I finally found my way in March of 2002 to a great doctor on Long Island, and began aggressive treatment for Babesia, Ehrlichia, Bartonella and Lyme. I had entered his office with the beginning symptoms of Parkinson's. I was petrified. I stuttered, my hands had tremors, one leg would drag, I drooled, I was scared out of my wits. Within two months of beginning treatment those symptoms were gone. It took another year and a half for the terrible encephalopathy headaches and associated depression to lessen. The fits of rage and my over reaction to stress were slowly disappearing. I have to say that is one of the worst symptoms of this disease, to know that you are going out of control and not be able to stop it. Again, family and individual therapy was sought, I did not want my daughter growing up with a mom like that. I cannot count how many times I have told her that my fits were not her fault, and that I was sorry I yelled at her.

Little by little, I began getting better. I woke up one day about a year into treatment, and "I" was back. I felt me again. I was afraid to move. I had a clear understanding at that point of how devastating this disease is, the depths that it drives us to, and how horrible it is emotionally. This feeling was to come and go, but slowly and with persistence on my doctor's part and mine for sticking with treatment, I have become much better.

I have had no brain fog since July 6, 2003. I am still in treatment and still continuing to get better. I have many parts of myself back, parts that I thought were gone forever. I am a different person, but I have a livable life, and can do many things although I am limited. I am grateful for what I have recovered and don't think I will ever take feeling good for granted again.

Its the hardest thing I have ever done, to secure and continue with treatment. People who I thought were friends thought I was faking, along with doctors and others. I avoided certain people, and then learned that life was better without them. Even one of my nurses pestered me continually, asking when I would be finished with treatment, and why didn't I go to one of the doctors in Boston if I wanted to get well. It finally dawned on me that I could ask for a more supportive nurse. May they never have to experience first-hand what its like to have Lyme and beg for treatment. Sometimes I felt almost criminal...guilty of something other than having a disease. Now I realize that is part of being ill, and a normal response to having been treated poorly, not only by some in the medical profession but by people I thought were friends. Needless to say, I have made adjustments in my life, and stayed with those who are supportive and helpful, who urged me to stick with treatment and hang on, things would get better. I have developed a strong faith, that which comes with the feeling of facing death.

I have survived the darkest depressions that are really like none I could ever imagine.. These came with the terrible headaches and pain that ran throughout every nerve in my body. There was very little relief available. I would lie in bed for days waiting for it to pass. I learned to enjoy and appreciate the days when I did feel good.

I have dealt with all that treatment brings. I have had the wrong diagnosis, the wrong doctors, doctors that quit, doctors that said very unintelligent or cruel things. One got very mad at me for having a PICC line order from my LLMD, and treated me with contempt afterwards. I have also met some wonderful dedicated doctors and have come to fully appreciate them and the roll that nurses play.

I have had sensitivities and allergies to drugs. I have had two friends die, one very close to me. (Neither from Lyme but both of them had it.) I have endured humiliating remarks and intrusive questions from all sorts of people. I have had doctors deny a first monitored dose of an IV drug at the infusion room at the hospital. I have had to deal with broken PICC lines.. I have been yelled at by many and varied medical practitioners, listened to them call my daughter and I names, refuse treatment, refuse to order tests, refuse to give the results of tests, and several who have walked out of exam rooms when the word Lyme is mentioned. I have lived through the deep dark fear of what I call "The Disease of a Thousand Deaths."

I have had to face the worst thoughts that a person can have and come to terms with it. I have put myself in the hospital more than once to stay safe.

I have had to take out loans to pay for tens of thousands of dollars for treatment, testing and non-covered medical items and drugs for my daughter and I. We have gone through six doctors in the process of being treated. None of this is unusual for a" Lymie." In fact, I consider myself lucky in light of what many others have gone through. I have gained some terrific and strong friends who have been there with me throughout each step. My parents and other family members have been very supportive. I have many times said I would rather give birth to an elephant than to have Lyme, at least then I would have a pet.

At some point I began to learn more about this disease, and have come to believe that it far surpasses any other infectious disease in its distribution and affect upon people. I believe it is a global epidemic and we as a nation are in near total denial of its rate of infection and impact on us. I also believe this is not a true and total act of nature but one that has been designed to infect and disable a large section of the population. The huge number of previously rare disorders that previously strike people in their adult hood are now impacting childhood and early adult years is frightening. Untreated Lyme mimics many other diseases and I believe it is grossly misdiagnosed as Lupus, MS, CFS and CFIDS, ALS, Alzheimer's, Parkinson's and other auto immune diseases. I believe it is the root cause of many psychological disorders. I further believe that it contributes greatly to the rate of violent crime in this country, and for the epidemic of suicide among teens.

In 2003, two friends and I began a chapter of one of the national organizations that has been so helpful in bringing about awareness of this disease and supporting the doctors who treat Lyme and the co-infections. We have done our best to help others find diagnosis, doctors and treatment, no easy task when we are trying to recover ourselves.

I also began cartooning as a way of processing and digesting what has happened to me. As an artist, I have found this avenue of creating easy to fit into the daily schedule of living with Lyme. I have found this very healing. I can only make light of that which I have been through. I have always, with the exception of a few dark times, relied on my sense of humor to see me through the worst. During the darkest days, I relied on others. In my very worst times, my faith. At times, I asked for a painless quick death. During the better times, I had to laugh at the irony of it all: A person once on the brink of death in a coma, who now very much wishes to live, and to live well. After all, isn't that the best revenge?

Looking back, nothing in my life compares to the depression, rage, loss, and pain of this disease. Others have said better than I can what insights they have gained from illness. It has changed my life completely, but given me a measure of compassion, an extension of understanding, some wonderful friends, a deep respect for the doctors that treat it, and a profound belief in the power of hope.

Chapter XII

Am I Invisible?

Carol's Story

Unlike some, I vividly remember my tick experience. I 1974, I was 12 years old and I found a little tiny mouse in a chicken coupe while out with my father. I scooped it up and proceeded to "raise" it as a pet, despite my father's insistence that I get rid of that thing!

I kept it hidden in a match box in my room and fed it with an eye dropper for weeks. After its eyes opened, it grew quickly. I remember lying on my bed and letting it run threw my hair! What on earth was I thinking? It grew quickly and I had to let it go. As if this wasn't bad enough, before I released it, it bit me.

In a recent discussion with my mom about my past health problems, it occurred to us that around the time of the mouse, I was also diagnosed with a case of "ring worm". A circular rash appeared on my ankle. My mother presumed I got it while running around barefoot in the chicken coups. The MD gave me a cream and it eventually went away. After looking at the photos of the "bulls eye rash," it's very possible that it wasn't ring worm after all! But, I never want to go near a chicken coup again as long as I live!

A few weeks after letting the mouse go, I woke up with a headache and felt weak. I told my mom I had a headache and didn't want to go to school. She started screaming at me, "I'm sick of this! Every time I tell you to do the dishes or go to school, you get a headache. That's it!! I'm taking you to the doctor!"

She thought this would provoke an instant recovery and I'd get ready for school. I told her I would go, but I was beginning to get weak and couldn't dress myself. She phoned the physician and insisted on a same-day appointment. When the doctor saw me, he honestly admitted to my mother that he had no clue what was wrong with me. He sent us to St. Catherine's in Hammond for an EEG.

On the way to St. Catherine's my neck became stiff and I began throwing up every five minutes. By the time I got to the hospital I could no longer walk and my father had to carry me in. I only remember bits and pieces of this day.

My mother and father have filled in the missing information. St. Catherine's staff was baffled as well, but completely certain that I was in trouble and referred us to Children's Memorial Hospital in Chicago, IL. My father, who used to be a taxi driver, got me there as quickly as possible.

When we got there a team of psychiatrists began asking me questions like, "do you love your mother?" My mother and father were frightened they were going to let me die while asking questions! Suddenly, a female doctor burst through the door and bellowed, "Has anyone bothered to give this child a spinal tap?" The room went silent and she ordered them to get out!

Within minutes I was getting my first spinal tap. I was told that my spinal fluid was so thick with infection that it was difficult to get out. I was soon admitted into Chicago's Children's Memorial Hospital with a diagnosis of spinal meningitis and encephalitis.

While in a coma, or "out of my mind" with fever, whatever you want to call it, I had hallucinations about grape bubble gum being under my bed. I refused to keep any clothes on. My mother told me that I had no modesty. Even when the preacher came to visit, I kept stripping my gown off in his presence.

I was packed in ice and put on a special COLD MAT that froze me something fierce. When the fever finally broke, I swore that I jumped out of the bed and turned the knob on the machine to

HOT and that's why I got better. (Despite the fact that I was out of it so long that I could no longer walk, much less get out of the bed). My mother found a fully engorged deer tick on my head while trying to remove EEG glue from my hair. My mother screamed for a nurse and things got crazy! They were scared to death and had no clue how to get it off. They pulled and pinched, to no avail. It was firmly planted in my head. Finally, some nurses came in with a book of matches and removed the tick. Nothing else was ever said about it to our family. No follow-up for the bite was ever done. I had therapy to learn to walk again and was released after a twelve-day stay.

After coming home from the hospital I suffered with severe headaches and couldn't stand upright for many months without severe blinding pain in my eyes. My left eye drooped from then on, especially when having a migraine headache, and I was told it was called a "lazy eye". I had to walk stooped over to prevent the blinding pains to my head and eyes. When I had a headache, all I could think about was ending the pain. The same is to this day. I don't like to be tortured or aggravated in any way. When the pain is at maximum, I will scream or do anything to get whatever is annoying me, away from me. I find that I basically have no control over my emotional reactions when I'm in that much pain, I just SNAP when things get too intense for me. I literally feel like I am losing my mind when I have a violent migraine.

I began to develop and my parents assumed the changes I was going through were because of being a teenager. I remember trying to explain to them that I felt funny since the hospital, and my mom threw a fit and said I blamed everything on being sick and that I was a hypochondriac ...blah, blah, blah... I'm not sure if this has any significance, but when I went to the hospital, I didn't have boobs. When I came home from the hospital, I needed a bra. In two weeks my chest grew that much. Despite that change, I did not start my period until I was nearly 16 years old.

When I got my license my parents bought me a 1974 blue Ford Maverick. I had it less than a month and I rolled it on a gravel road. Things just got worse, as I went from being a straight "A" student to a "C-F" student. My previous activities of twirling and acrobats had to be discontinued as I could not bend over or stand up without dizziness and pain. I still had migraine headaches even with very little activity. I became more inactive and gained some weight.

I missed at least three days of school per month. The PMS was crazy! I'd be so violent and upset without a clue it was coming.

I couldn't think or function. Of course, this just set my mother off even further. She said all women had periods and I was overacting to get attention! I grew distant from my family, quit school and left home at age sixteen. I went through three husbands and ended up back at home with my mother.

Over the years I've suffered with SEVERE menstrual difficulties, SEVERE migraines, SEVERE fatigue, obsessive/compulsive behavior, AGGRESSIVENESS, moodiness & crying spells, weight gain, poor balance, frequent ear infections and upper chest infections, bronchitis, tonsillitis. SEVERE knee/foot joint pain (four surgeries on right foot alone), EXTREMELY slow healer, VERY touchy skin (hurts all the time and adhesive or even Band-Aids irritate and breaks down my skin very quickly) normal body temp of 97.1-97.7 degrees, loud snoring, apnea, insomnia, sleep problems, major intolerance to heat/cold, allergies, left trapezoidal muscle and neck pain, rib cage pain, muscle weakness, tingling in my hands and feet and shortness of breath. Another thing, I get really weak, irritated, and nauseous and get a headache if I'm food or sleep deprived for too long.

I just knew if I could get out of the house and away from my mother that things would be better. The peace of mind of being away from her did wonders. Except my new husband didn't know how to deal with my menstrual mania either. He began to get physically abusive and I responded in like fashion.

I landed a good job at an insurance company and we started attending church. I desperately wanted a child, thinking that's what my life needed. After about six months of trying I became pregnant with my daughter. From 1980-83 I worked in an office position. I fell once and had another car wreck. Neck pain, headaches and fatigue accompanied the pregnancy and were thought to be a part of the process.

I was 20 years old when she was born on November 8, 1981. I wanted to be a good mother so I decided to breast feed. My daughter was extremely colicky. I sought help from breast-feeding experts, who claimed my milk had to be good for my baby. I watched everything I ate and my daughter continued to cry. After five weeks of my daughter's continuous crying, my mother offered to take her for a night to give me some rest. My mom violated my wishes and fed her formula instead of my pumped milk as I asked her to. My daughter slept through the night for the first time after getting formula instead of my milk. I was so hurt that my milk made her sick. She became a completely different child after that. What a happy, content little joy she was! I felt guilty over that for a long time.

I began developing allergies that I never had before. I began having major problems completing tasks. Mood swings became more apparent. I began having increased problems getting along with others. I had no ability to handle stress at all. I began reading self-help books and tried every diet imaginable in an effort to make my life better. In 1983, the company was in the process of closing the office and I left my job because I couldn't handle the stress of the situation.

I was 23 years old when I first stepped into a bar. Of course, I drank and partied like an idiot. And this is when I learned of my intolerance of alcohol. I got drunk easily. It also caused severe headaches and though I have a social drink now and then, I really don't care for it to this day.

Not long after getting to North Carolina, I got very ill. The stress of new job began to take its toll. I came down with MONO, URI, Bronchitis, and Tonsillitis and was told that my kidneys were possibly slightly damaged by the infection. After two weeks in bed I tried to go back to work. But I was slower and my boss was angry about frequent misfiled documents. I had another bad car wreck on a blind curve and hit a dirt embankment. The car rolled on its side and I don't remember anything until a fireman slapped me in an attempt to get me to stop screaming "where's my daughter", who by the way, was sitting on my lap. I have no clue how I got out of the car, how long we were there, etc. I went home and was down another two weeks with severe headaches and neck stiffness. A chiropractor drained all of my insurance benefits claiming to help me. I didn't get any better for a long time and couldn't work. I lost my job and had to move home with my parents.

The only drug that ever really helped was Fiorcet. My aunt had severe migraines, good insurance and was referred to the Diamond Headache Clinic. So when they tried it on her and it worked, she told me. I told my doctor, and he let me try it. To my surprise and delight it really helped. I was finally able to stop the headache instead of having to live through them!

In 1986, I married my childhood sweetheart. In 1987, I was pregnant with my son, and again gained an unusually large amount of weight. The only excuse I have is that I was sick at my stomach all the time unless there was food in it.

My son was born with a strange condition. When he got angry, upset, or scared he would become unable to breathe, turn blue, and pass out. Later down the road he would shake violently if you scolded him. The doctor told us to just let him lay there and he would breathe on his own. It was a frightening time for us. Again, this was during a time when we had no insurance available to us, so further testing was not an option.

In 1986, I had trained to be a CNA/HHA and began doing home health for private agencies and would continue to do so for the next nine years. This allowed me to make my own schedule so I could work around my constant illnesses.

For example, I knew I would wake up with a headache every day, so I didn't schedule morning clients. I'd get up, take a Fiorcet, and get the pain under control and do my first client at 10:00am. The shifts were only 2 hours long and entailed helping Medicare patients bathe among other things. Even if I were in poor shape during a visit, I could usually pull it off. This is how I was able to be employed while ill for all those years.

In 1991 my husband died suddenly in an automobile accident. I also lost eight other family members and friends during a 9 month period. I was instantly and completely disabled. I began having severe panic attacks and hallucinations. Night terror and nightmares were also common. Fatigue and a deep fog came over me. I lost my job. I gained massive amounts of weight. Mood swings were common. I was very abusive to my oldest child. For about three years I was totally not myself. I have very few memories. It's like one long black out to me. I'm told I cried constantly and my daughter called for delivered food to feed us and helped care for her brother.

The problem of me snapping came out at it's worst at this point in my life. I wouldn't realize I had PMS coming on, and I'd just fly into a rage. The worse the stress was, the worse the rage would be. I saw an MD who said I had all the signs of Chronic Fatigue Syndrome. Another told me Candida, and the list goes on to include, Fibromyalgia, Depression, Over-weight, Stress, just to name a few. I'll be the first to admit that I'd feel better if I lost weight. But, you'll have to admit, it's very difficult to exercise when every time you bend over or turn your head it swims.

A few blaring facts stand out to me: 1) the majority of my pains were centered in the left side of my head/eye, the back of my neck, and my left shoulder. 2) I seem to always have some kind of infection going on, i.e. eyes, ears, sinuses, URI, etc. 3) My knees and feet had begun to hurt severely also. My feet felt like they were on FIRE. They hurt like no pain I had ever known before and have continued to be a major issue to this day, second only to my headaches and menstrual difficulties.

I wanted badly to find help. I had no job, no insurance and no one to turn to. I just did the best I could to keep it under control. My mother could see I was not in good shape and her idea of helping the situation was to threaten to take my kids away every time she saw me. In response to her threats I distanced myself from everyone to keep my problems under wrap because my kids were my "everything." And though I knew I desperately needed help, I would never let anyone take them away from me!

Eventually, I was placed on 40mg of Valium per day to shut me up. This therapy was only making matters worse for me, so I started weaning myself the medication. The horrible, blinding headaches continued. Once I got off the Valium I saw a massage therapist who helped to relax me and get my blood flowing and I began exercising a very little at a time. Between the massages and the Fiorcet, I was able to find a little relief. Not quality of life, just relief.

Around 1993, I started to feel a little better. I continued to have many of the same symptoms and I was still very slow compared to my previous self. I married again. He was looking for a place to stay and I needed help. In the early dating months I helped him to land a good job using my secretarial skills to write resumes and make phone calls for him. Once he landed the job, he and I married so I could use his insurance to try and get better. We claimed to love each other at the time, but in my heart I know I was desperate and willing to try anything to get better.

I remember I had severe sinus infections and swollen glands all the time and on antibiotics every time I turned around. Each time I pursued my medical issues with an MD (being sure to mention the tick), he would give me another physical and a few blood tests and tell me I was fine.

I can't quite remember when/where/who about which doctor I was seeing at the time, but at one point in my attempts to get treatment after a blood test, I was told by a physician that I had to redo a blood test, and if it didn't come back any better, I would definitely need a kidney specialist. The test came back with better results and those are the only times I can remember when my kidney function was in question.

When I told them I don't feel fine. Something doesn't feel fine in my head, they would get that "oh you need a psychiatrist" look in their eyes and offer me Prozac. You can only imagine the type of mother and wife I was despite my best efforts. I tried so hard not to be a burden, but I was always ill.

In 1994, I tried to return to the work world. After one month on the job, the left shoulder trapezoidal muscle group was "pulled" and I was sent to the University of Chicago with many of the same complaints that I have now.
(Dizziness, poor balance, headaches, fatigue, pain in my neck, shoulder and ears.) They did a test where they make lights go real fast in front of my eyes, and then they squirted water in my ears. I got very nauseous and never received any results from the test. I continued to have frequent over-whelming migraine headaches. About every couple of months I'd end up in the ER with a migraine I couldn't control. They'd shoot me up with Demerol and I'd get over it in a few hours and go home to sleep a couple of days. Eventually I was referred to a pain clinic, where I was shot up with steroids about my neck and shoulders. This would always be followed by weight gain, inactivity and flu-like symptoms. All my problems were blamed on being over-weight, large breasts and depression. Once again, I was told
that there was nothing wrong with me.

In 1996, I fell down going out the front door of our house. This accident brought on increased inactivity and migraine headaches. Naturally my husband and I began to have major problems. He became terribly abusive in response to my constant illness. The marriage ended in 1997. I began working at McDonalds in an attempt to support myself and children. After a few months there, I slipped on a wet floor. My ankle and foot hyper-extended when I slipped, but did I didn't fall down. From that point on I had balance problems and started falling over on a regular basis. In an attempt to appease the insurance company and avoid surgery it was necessary to receive steroid injections. After three tries I was finally referred to a specialist who deemed the surgery necessary. I was told the ligament ripped off the bone in my ankle. It was surgically repaired and just would not heal. The tissue around the incision was irritated and five weeks later I developed a mysterious post-surgical infection. I was placed on several different intravenous antibiotics which didn't work. The infection had to be surgically removed from my ankle. My veins, like my skin were very irritated and the IV lines would blow daily. Each day they had to find a new site to stick a new IV line in and eventually a PIC-line had to be surgically inserted to my heart. I kept the line in for nine weeks. During this time I was too weak to walk and spent several months in a wheel chair.

Within 24 hours of pulling the PIC-line my entire head became infected "mysteriously" and I was back in the hospital once again. I was tested for a lot of stuff including AIDS, but the infectious disease specialist refused to test for Lyme, as it **wasn't possible**. I could not tolerate any light. My head hurt like never before. And I was placed back on intravenous Vancomycin along with Morphine this time due to the severe pain. After five days in the hospital, the infection was brought under control once again, and I was sent home on oral antibiotics. Here's the crazy part. Upon finally healing up, I felt better than **ever** before.

In 1998, I lost 50 lbs.; was accepted by Purdue University College; landed a tool & die apprenticeship in a stamping plant; was able to buy a car and place of my own; got on the Dean's list and accepted into the National Scholar's Honor Society; and started working on a bachelor's degree in Industrial Engineering Technologies...My life was finally coming together.

I was still a little forgetful and I had to really study my butt off. Student support services helped me to use tutors for math, but I could do it! For the first time since I was a little girl my parents were seeing the old me and they were proud of me! My family and I began repairing our relationships. All this after being treated just one long-term time with intravenous antibiotics I found out what it's like to live nearly symptom free and it was wonderful. I was finally able to support myself and I liked it. It was short-lived, but it was the happiest time of my life. I was so happy and proud of myself. I could think more clearly and started making new friends. It was like someone walked into my head and turned on the lights. And now that I am aware of Lyme disease, this is why I believe antibiotic treatment works on Third Stage Chronic Lyme.

Though I don't doubt my perceptions of certain people's feelings toward me, I fear I may embellish situations with my overwhelming paranoia at certain points, making matters worse. I shake inside all the time. My injuries and accidents continued. While on top of a piece of equipment at work in late 1998, I fell and jammed my knees and shoulders on solid steel. This started the knee and shoulder complaints I still suffer with today. I was told by a workman's compensation doctor that I have arthritis. Moist heat treatments helped the most. Ibuprofen made it possible for me to continue to work. I was given physical therapy three times a week and placed on light duty. During this time, I experienced increased migraines. It took a long time to heal, but I finally got back on the job. I could tell I was really beginning to slow down at a fast rate. I was working full time and attending college in the evenings. I hadn't been able to do anything for so long, but I wanted to do it all now.

Not long after, during a stressful situation I came down with shingles and missed work for 14 days. This was followed by numerous head/sinus/inner ear infections that kept me out of work and on antibiotics for weeks at a time.

Later in 1999, I injured my neck/shoulder again. This time I was pulling a large fan and the pain just hit me. The next day I couldn't lift my left arm and I experience severe neck and head pain. The doctor repeated the treatment he had when I had jammed my knees. Eventually they sent me to a specialist who evaluated me for possible Thorastic Outlet Syndrome because of the tingling and gloved feeling I was experiencing in my hands. I had an EMG and was told there was no blood flow problem with my arms. My hands and arms continue to tingle today, especially when I lie down to sleep. Still, no one could find a problem, so it was determined that I have arthritis or bursitis in my shoulders too.

Somewhere along the lines of my treatment, I got an MRI and found out that I have a brain malformation. Soon, I had to have another surgery. After starting my apprenticeship I began to have breakthrough bleeding. By early 1999 I began having two periods a month. In the fall of 1999 I bled for 3 months straight, from another mystery infection, this time, in my uterus. On January 4, 2000, I finally got a complete hysterectomy. One of the happiest days of my life. The doctor said my uterus was the size of someone about six months pregnant; I had endometriosis, adomyosis (which was described to me as endometriosis in the lining of the uterus, again irritated tissue), fibroid tumors, and scars on my ovaries. Of all my suffering, the migraines and abdominal pain of my cycle were the worst. After the surgery I continued to bleed (tissue at incision was irritated and would not heal externally or internally) and had to be internally cauterized with silver nitrate for nine weeks straight. It took 8 months and physical therapy for me to return to work from the surgery. The migraine headaches decreased as a result and I was able to exercise a little bit more.

Not long after returning to work in the fall of 2001, I tripped over a piece of steel and crashed to the floor. The trauma of the fall seemed to trigger the previous symptoms and more. Every joint in my body hurt. My balance was gone once again. And my migraines which had been mostly under control since my hysterectomy in 2000, suddenly reoccurred. I was on light duty and in therapy for most of 2001.

Then while driving home from work in February 2002, I wrecked my truck. I don't know what I hit. I was in a dream- like state and have no idea what really happened. Three months later, on June 1, 2002, I fell fifteen feet down a flight of stairs. I was walking, and then my feet wouldn't move. The next thing I knew I was cart-wheeling through the air to the bottom of the stairs. I figured the reason I fell must be my foot and knee from the fall at work. I broke my left ankle (the good one!!!), got whiplash, a concussion and multiple contusions and bruises about my body. My right knee, right arm and forehead had very deep, large bruises that took forever to heal. This is when I got the worst I've ever been.

On December 16, 2002, I finally had surgery on my right foot, as previously scheduled prior to the big fall down the stairs. The joint was packed full of infection (Another mystery infection) and part of the bone was dissolved. Tests of the removed tissue showed no cancer. Once I was able to walk, I was ready to begin therapy. I requested that my PCP allow therapy for my neck/arms/shoulders as I was still experiencing problems. He questioned the fact that I had taken so long to seek treatment. I explained that I was on the "traditional insurance plan" from work, which meant I was responsible for paying the office calls. Plus, Ford's National Foot Care program was messing with my treatment, which slowed down the approval of my surgery. And most importantly, since the fall I am experiencing confusion. When I tried to take on more appointments and MD's I became over-whelmed and had to focus on one thing at a time. In my heart, I truly hoped that my head, which is still dented where I hit it in the fall, would snap out of it. But it hasn't. Even my handwriting and typing skills are affected!

After falling down the stairs, something drastically changed in my head. I could no longer keep up with my paperwork at home. I began stuffing my bills into bags because I couldn't deal with them. My checks bounced. My phone/cable/etc. would get cut off. I lost my car keys so much I had to begin tying them to the door knob as soon as I came in or I'd spend hours looking for them later. I would make lists, and in the morning I couldn't remember where I put the lists. People would have conversations with me one day and the next day, I could not recall seeing them much less the conversation.

I remember going to the mall and walking with someone I've known for years, and I looked at them, and couldn't recall their name! I would get in my car to go someplace and either not know how I got there or forget where I was going. I began falling asleep at the wheel regularly, especially at night or in bright sunlight. That's another thing, I can barely stand being in the sun or bright lights. I'd start to pull out and a car would just appear. This is when I began staying home alone, A LOT. I still do. I don't like being dizzy, as it makes me nauseous. I socially withdrew from my friends to avoid the embarrassment of frequent verbal mistakes during conversations. I hardly see anyone, except the neighbor next door. I'm too dizzy to enjoy our nightly walks anymore, but she still comes by to visit.

Despite all the slack I received from my professors, thanks to Student Support Services, I still had to drop my classes, the semester following the fall. I requested a medical note explaining my circumstances as I had a fabulous two-year grant that I didn't want to lose!

I told the PCP, there's something wrong inside my head. I can't even do math now when I had received an "A" in my last trig class! The attending PCP stated he wouldn't write me a note unless I saw a neurologist. He gave me a referral and I made the appointment. I began to think he didn't believe I was ill.   My daughter went to these appointments with me and was very upset about the MD's attitude also. Fortunately, my reputation for being a good student bought me the slack I needed to keep my grant. No thanks to that JERK of a doctor. I dropped all but one of the classes and tried to concentrate on getting well.

In the meantime, my PCP allowed me to receive therapy for my neck/shoulders in addition to my foot following surgery. During therapy of my neck/shoulders I experienced extreme pain in my neck and the left shoulder/trapezoidal area. Working the neck/shoulder area, my migraine headaches became more frequent and intense. After only a few appointments, I had to discontinue therapy of the neck and shoulder because it was too painful and the headaches were out of control.

I began to pursue the headache issue with a neurologist, as it was the symptom keeping me down the most. The neurologist placed me on Topomax to help prevent the headaches and ordered an EEG and MRI's of my head and neck area. The Topomax worked on the headaches, but the dizziness/confusion/memory problems became more apparent.

Today my neck is stiff and hurts all the time. My left shoulder pain is back. My rib cage pain is back. I'm disoriented, spaced-out, and unable to complete simple tasks. Paying bills or messing with paperwork always ends in disaster for me.

Through my research on the Web I had found that not only do the symptoms I've been suffering with for some time line up with the Lyme issue, but that the diagnosis of Lyme disease is "CLINICAL", and many times cannot be defined by blood testing. Many times, especially Third Stage Lyme Disease patients, rarely get positive blood test results, as the disease hides deeply in the cells. I also found documentation that explains why I got so much worse after the fall. People who suffer a concussion, as I did in the fall, can get a post-concussion syndrome that sparks the disease to present increased symptoms and "wake up" or encourage Lyme symptoms.

Now this all began to make sense!

I researched on-line as much as my eyes would allow, and began writing my history down, as much as I could remember. I interviewed both my parents to fill in the blanks. The IV treatment I received in 1997 explains why I was in such great shape after the post-surgical infection.

After the fall, my eyesight immediately worsened by more than twice. The headaches returned much worse and became out of control. X-rays of my knees revealed joint deterioration there also. Not only do my injuries/accidents continue, but they are becoming more frequent.

Another sinus and UTI infection, requiring three different antibiotics, brought me back to my doctor. He also put me on a steroidal nasal spray. Each time I took antibiotics I got sicker. I told the MD that the antibiotics just weren't working because I was getting sicker; he'd try another one. I wasn't aware of the Herheimer reaction at the time, or I would have known what was going on.

After seeing the neurologist again with my history, he asked if I had been tested for Lyme disease. Of course, I said no because I had been told that it couldn't be. He said he would check for it anyway. He prescribed ordered some blood tests (including Lyme Disease). I was overjoyed that he was being so thorough. I went home and looked up all kinds of info on the internet and got the SHOCK of my life. I found out that Lyme can be forever to those who didn't receive treatment at the time of infection.

I attempted to return to work in April 2003. I was only able to work half days due to fatigue and pain, not to mention, it was very apparent that the noise of the plant was adding to my dizziness and confusion. I worked four days, took some vacation time I had coming and contacted the neurologist again. After insisting that it had been long enough (20 days) since the tests had been done, he finally read the tests. He called me on the phone the following day.

The EEG was abnormal showing a possibility of seizures. The MRI's showed spots on my brain. I have an Arnold Chirari brain malformation and enlarged ventricles in my brain. He referred me to an infectious disease specialist to further investigate the Lyme issue. He blatantly stated that he had no knowledge of Lyme disease, nor did he want to have any knowledge of it. He went on to explain that I had been born with an Arnold Kuari brain malformation and the ventricles in my brain are enlarged, which will cause headaches. I have spots on my brain and an abnormal EEG which shows I may be having petite mall seizures and would account for my frequent falls and driving experience. He took away my driving privileges and put me on a stronger seizure medication.

I explained that I knew of the malformation (which just means that the lower lobe of my brain is situated in my head a little lower than most) and that I'd been told it was no big deal/non-symptomatic years ago. As for the spots, they could be from my fall or Lyme damage.

I had done my homework and took several key pieces of Lyme information, including a three-page personal history that took me five days to type due to my memory and attention span problems. The Neurologist was so rude and refused the papers I offered. He kept asking questions that were already answered in the paper I just handed him. I told him, I wrote it down because when I try to tell anyone anything, I become confused.

Things just got uglier and long story kept short, he is no longer my neurologist. I've been referred to infectious disease specialist (with orders to rule out Lyme). Whether that will do me any good or not, I don't know.

What a shame to see a medical professional behave in such a manner. And just for the record, I was on my "best behavior" when I was there. For one thing I was just too sick to cause much trouble. He acted like he was sitting there with a loaded gun, just waiting for me to walk in the door.

My Lyme test was negative, but said that he had other plans. I'm not sure what all he was talking about, but I remember, hospital, dye, spine, and shunt... All I know is nobody is cutting on me until my blood test results come back from New Jersey. And from what I've read, it may take several attempts or different types of tests to find a Lyme bug as they are very tricky to catch. Generally Lyme diagnosis and treatment begins with a "clinical" diagnosis.

I signed up for college classes this semester again in order to keep the previously mentioned grant. I had to drop Chemistry early on. The extensive reports required, in addition to the mathematical requirements, were too difficult for me to handle. My reading/typing/math skills have all gone to hell since the fall. I missed a large portion of this semester's classes due to migraines, fatigue and "flu". (At least that's what my PCP was calling it.) Then when I attempted to return to work and started having much worse dizziness, I had to throw in the towel.

For all these years I've listened to doctors tell me it can't be LYME, while I suffer bizarre symptoms. Then amazingly when I did get treated with intravenous antibiotics (the initial method of treatment for Lyme disease) my life completely turned around.

I cried a river of tears and screamed until I had no voice, when my mother told me that they didn't give me any antibiotics when I was in the hospital in 1974, as they felt the infection must have been viral. In the meantime, negative Lyme test results came back from the Indiana lab.

I had already gotten on-line and asked a few questions. A lady from Texas told me of a person, who lives nearby me, that has Lyme and started a local Lyme support group. She explained to me that Indiana labs are not finding the Lyme as their testing techniques are not up to par for finding the bug.

To my understanding the Lyme test they ran checked my body for the antibodies to Lyme disease, and may not be present due to the way antibiotics work on Lyme. They create a "hostile environment" that causes the organism to become temporarily dormant. Most if not all antibiotics can accomplish this, although obviously some are more effective than others, and some penetrate various tissues better than others.

The "cyst" form of Lyme is a form the actual spirochete takes to hide from antibiotics or other threatening agents. The spirochete... a cork screw shaped bacterium that does that evolving thingy and only the strong survive thingy... ends up in a coated protective ball and "hides" to survive.

According to a prominent Lyme specialist in New York, Vancomycin is the best antibiotic for treating resistant strains of Lyme. It is also the best antibiotic for penetrating the tissues in the brain/head. You can't deny the possibility that I may have gotten better in 1997, because the Vancomycin addressed the Lyme infection in my head.

The support group leader helped me to find a Lyme disease Literate Nurse Practitioner, (LDL NP) who is currently treating 67 Lyme patients from the area. The doctor put me on 200mg of Doxycyline per day and sent my blood to both CA and NJ for appropriate DNA testing.

On the 4th day of being on Doxycyline I started running a fever and my right ear became infected. My skin started hurting worse and I had chills and night sweats. My neck became stiff. My left shoulder kicked up in miserable pain. My sinuses had pressure and my head hurt. It pretty much felt like I had a bad case of the flu. These symptoms indicated a "JARISCH HERXHEIMER REACTION," due to the antibiotics; which is another strong indication of Lyme disease.

On the 10th day of taking the antibiotic, the symptoms started to ease up some. I wasn't as hot and my skin felt better. I began taking in fluids and food. The headaches had backed off. Though the symptoms continue to come and go, I stayed on the Doxycyline 200mg per day. I stopped taking the Doxycyline when I became extremely ill and unable to function on May 1, 2003. I also stopped taking the Trileptal from the neurologist. I have not started taking the Topomax again either. There were just too many new medications and symptoms for me to sort it out and I was frightened. I want to wait until I receive an opinion from the specialist in MO on how to proceed from here.

So, that's my story. I strongly feel I have at least one, and more than likely multiple, tick borne disease in my blood. I plan to pursue that to the fullest extent. I refuse to believe that all these things that have happened to me are just coincidences any further.

I'm not out and out rejecting any other physician's opinion of my state of health. Obviously, I have serious concerns in my brain according to the recent test results. I just believe that after all I've been through; I deserve the opportunity to FIND out once and for all if treatment for Lyme will indeed help me again. I can't stay like this... not after tasting what a REAL life is like!

Furthermore, it is a FACT that people with Lyme disease have the exact same symptoms as I've been experiencing for nearly 30 years; and after treatment the tissues in their brains heal; EEG's become normal and their symptoms subside. Just like mine did after the antibiotic treatment in 1997.

As a matter of post-thought, I strongly believe that IF I'd have had the ability to stay with ONE physician over the years, I think he/she would have put this together. But because of my lack of insurance for all those years and the frequent HMO, MD changes I had after getting insurance, my records are all over the place and I rarely see the same MD for more than a year or two.

Lyme has been reported to have been found in every single state in the US. Lyme disease is known as the "great imitator." It is **frequently** misdiagnosed as Lupus, MS, Chronic Fatigue Syndrome, Fibromyalgia, Candida, etc. Please research the subject very carefully & thoughtfully before making allowing anyone to make a snap decision about your diagnosis. Did you know that there is no specific test to prove you have MS, Lupus or Chronic Fatigue Syndrome??

I began treatment with a Lyme literate MD on 5-14-03. Still suffering, but at least I know what I'm fighting now. Since beginning antibiotic therapy for Lyme Disease, I have been on a roller coaster of ups and downs. But it's better than doing nothing. I still fight my HMO for care daily. My HMO PCP refuses to honor most of my requests for referrals to appropriate specialists. My health has steadily gone down hill since my knee surgery. The dizziness and fatigue is taking over most of the time. Every now and then I experience a brief period of clarity. The only thing that stays the same is the fact that my symptoms change constantly.

I'd been begging for orthopedic care for months and when my right knee went out and I fell on Dec 16, 2004, I finally got the orthopedic referral, as my knee required surgery! Time after time this is how it goes for me. I have to be dying or severely injured to get medical attention!
At that time he also allowed the ophthalmologist referral I had been begging for after due to severe eye pain. The ophthalmologist found swollen optic nerves, Graves' disease, and strong indications of a pseudo tumor.

I requested a referral to see a pituitary specialist that works with my LLMD in January, 2004, to investigate the hormonal issues raised by the ophthalmologist appointment. Unfortunately, my PCP hasn't seen fit to respond or come up with a referral as usual. On Feb 2, 2004, I went on my own to see her. She contacted my PCP and received authorization to order a large hormone panel and I am awaiting the results. I have approached the state of Indiana on several levels with regard to the neglect and abuse I am being subjected to by MD's/HMO system that are not educated about Lyme disease.

I have asked the IN State's Attorney General to investigate my physicians and help me to receive the care I deserve. Because of the lack of understanding and necessary MD documentation of my Lyme illness, I was turned down by SSI disability AGAIN! I just had to file bankruptcy due to medical bills again!! This is a nightmare!!

I've written articles and faxed them to over 30 Indiana newspapers, and didn't get a kind word from one of them. I've spent hundreds of dollars on phone bills trying to bring attention to my plight. I attempted to turn the HMO in to the Insurance commissioner and found that my employer is self insured and I have to approach the IL Dept. of Labor for assistance.

After contacting the IL Dept of Labor, I was told that I would have to sue my employer for breach of contract to do anything about my lack of care. That all sounds so very wrong to me, but at the same time, it explains how I am being railroaded by the system and how they are getting away with it!!!

The bottom line is Indiana MD's have not been properly educated in the diagnosis and treatment of Lyme patients, esp. the 3rd stage. Most do not consider it unless a bulls eye rash is present at the time of examination, eliminating proper diagnosis and treatment for 85% of Lyme stricken patients right off the bat!

I have confronted my HMO/PCP with regard to the lack of appropriate care only to be ignored and shunned. I will not give up. I want to get well and I am tired of being invisible!

At last count, Carol has contacted a state congressman and rounded up support all over the country. She wants better care in Indiana and the insurance companies here to support treatment. The letters and calls that came into the Congressman's office came in so fast and furious that an aide called to ask that it all stop. He was responsible for answering these inquests and the job was mounting. Looks like we just might see Lyme Disease as a serious problem in Indiana. Way to go Carol!

CHAPTER XIII

I call it a MIRACLE

Ryan's Story

I approached my son's HMO pediatrician about testing for Lyme Disease. She reluctantly agreed to a titer test. I asked her about a WB instead as titers were useless. She opened a little book and told me that if the titer was negative, she'd look for another reason that Ryan's legs hurt and sleeping in class.

After the titer came back negative, I just decided to take him to Dr. C and forget about dealing with her. It was obvious that she didn't know a thing about Lyme Disease, nor did she care. She didn't have one tick poster on the wall and had the nerve to tell me that Ryan couldn't have gotten it from me unless the tick bite I got was in a certain TRIMESTER!?

Since then he has been diagnosed with Bb by Dr. C. I've been asking the school what type of assistance we could get to help him do better in school. I only knew of alternative school, and they insisted that he couldn't do it unless he worked. Well the kid is too tired to make it through a full day of school. I'm seriously doubting adding a job would be beneficial to the situation.

So, I tried to contact his school counselor and as usual she wasn't available. One of the other guidance counselors spoke to me and I explained that Ryan has an illness. He's on medications that make him not feel well and he has sleep difficulties. She proceeds to tell me they have a lot of kids on Doxy and he doesn't need special treatment for that.

I resisted the temptation to rip her tongue from her face, and told her that whether my son was getting ill or not was NOT in question. I am the parent and I just told you he IS ill and I'd like to know what we can do about it. She snarled back that she couldn't help me, but she'd give his counselor the message.

In the meantime, I got an e-mail from a gal on one of the Lyme Disease boards. She read an old post and stumbled onto my web page and contacted me out of the blue. We talked about our kids and their Lyme Disease. She said that she had a friend that had gone through the same thing regarding education. She offered to give me all the information she had on the subject and I gladly accepted.

Next, I called both the superintendents office and the principal, trying to find out what programs were available for my son. Of course neither could come to the phone, so I left more messages.

Finally, I get a call from the school counselor, who proceeds to blast me for calling around too much. She told me that the principal and the superintendent had thrown this in her lap to deal with. There was a lot of confusion and it was all my fault for putting my fingers in too many pies! She even had the nerve to tell me they have a chain of command that I was to follow! She said there is a 504 program, but she wouldn't discuss it with me or attempt to give me paperwork till I had a MD note stating Ryan has Lyme Disease. I told her the lab results just came back and the MD was in the process of doing just that.

I called the superintendent again and left her another message saying I was very upset to have her throw my inquiry "into someone else's lap" to deal with. I explained the resistance I was getting. She finally called back the next day and said she was sorry the counselor had been rude and she'd handle it. She also agreed to set up a meeting right away. I got the letter from Dr. C and a meeting was scheduled for the next morning.

That night, that lady's friend from the Lyme Disease board emailed me and we talked on the phone. She explained 504 plan vs. IEP. She coached me till we were both very sleepy. Then called me for another pep talk the following morning before I left for the school meeting. Plus she is helping me to find a "parent advocate" to keep the school from jacking me around.

In the meantime, the school counselor faxes me three pages, with no cover letter, regarding 504 plans that I guess she wanted filled out. The letter Dr. C sent covered all the questions, so I didn't bother with it. When I got to the meeting, the superintendent, the principal, my son's counselor and the school nurse were in attendance. The superintendent spoke first and said she wanted to proceed with a 504 plan for my son based upon the Dr. C's letter.

The school counselor said she had faxed papers to me and they couldn't proceed unless they were filled out. The superintendent read all the questions out loud and pulled the answers from the letter and said that this would do for now. We proceeded with the meeting.

While flames appeared to be shooting from the counselor's nose, she throws a piece of paper at me and says what about this? I looked at it. It was a fax from my son's old pediatrician. On her script pad was written, "Ryan does NOT have Lyme Disease. Negative Elisa test." And signed it. It was dated for the previous day. (The same day the superintendent reprimanded the counselor for being mean to me!) Can you spell Retaliation??

I asked her where she got that note, as I wasn't aware that it was a part of my son's medical record. I also explained that I hadn't signed any documents giving them permission to request any information from that MD, nor had I given that MD permission to share any info with them, as we weren't seeing that MD any more.

She looked all innocent like and said, I don't even know who your son's pediatrician is... it just showed up. No one in the room took responsibility for the inquiry.

I explained the situation about switching MD's over them not willing to test further or make clinical diagnosis. All the while I'm looking like a liar. The superintendent said that it was obvious from the letter provided by my son's specialist that he needed shortened days. She wanted to get started on the 504 plan.

I asked if I might speak. They said sure and I explained that Id been calling this school asking for guidance to assist my son with special needs. I was going to let my son quit or go to alternative school in desperation. Then I finally found out about the 504 plan and get here for the meeting. And so far, no one had even mentioned an IEP (Individual Education Plan) for my son.

I was feeling defensive and distrustful as they, a school system, hadn't given me complete information when I asked for it. My son has rights and he is entitle to a FREE battery of tests and accommodations to facilitate quality education to meet his needs.

I also stated that the counselor seemed to be very negative and unwilling to help us. I asked for an explanation.

The room was totally silent and they looked around at each other. Finally the superintendent spoke up and said that they didn't have an excuse, but that they would like to help. She said this needed to be a constructive meeting and suggested we all go forward from here. They admitted that they could test him for an IEP, but wanted to start with a 504 based on Dr. C's letter.

The superintendent suggested shortened days for Ryan's fatigue. He is going to get a bus at 12 noon (instead of 7:00am) and stay to the usual 3:15pm allowing him to rest more at home. In addition, she suggested the school give him a laptop (that was made for that purpose and available at the time) with the assignments on it so he could work more from home.

Needless to say I was VERY happy with that. Then after testing, which they have 60 "school days" to render, we'll work on his IEP. Also, since I'm ordered by my MD to not drive, our future meetings will be done by phone conference.

While taking the testing application, it was noted that my MD was in MO and he said that may be a problem as the process requires an INDIANA MD. I said and if you have a kid with cancer who goes to MAYO for treatment do you do the same to them.

After making the testing application, the counselor was to help me set up his new schedule. Instead she wanted to whine about not having her three pages filled out. She and I talked for quite a while. I told her I'd get the papers for her. We agreed on a tentative plan. Before leaving I looked her in the eye and said, "look, I'm upset and worried about my child. If in any way I've offended you, I'd like to bury the hatchet and start a new for my son's sake." She looked me dead in the eye while shaking my hand and swore to me that she had nothing to do with the "note" from Ryan's old MD. I accepted that and left.

I couldn't beat feet to the phone fast enough when I got home to call the MD's office. Sure enough, the counselor who just swore to me she had nothing to do with getting the note from the previous doctor was, in fact, the one who had requested the note on the school's behalf! Furthermore, the doctor created and faxed the document for her WITHOUT my permission! I told the MD's office that I had signed a new law form that stated it was ILLEGAL for a doctor's office to send medical records regarding any patient to a party without WRITTEN PERMISSION. Furthermore my son is a minor child. She faxed me the copy of the message taken when the counselor called and gave a message to the office coordinator.

I called the principal, but he was too busy to come to the phone. So I called superintendent's office again. She took my call and I reminded her of the situation with the MYSTERIOUS MD note that appeared in the meeting. She acknowledged that she remembered the incident. I proceeded to tell her how the counselor did do it and I had proof. The law had been broken. My son was being discriminated against because he had Lyme Disease and that my next phone call was to a special education civil rights lawyer.

She said she was shocked. She had nothing to do with the deceit. She asked that I fax her the proof right away and she was on her way to the school right then.

About a half an hour later the principal returned my call. (Oh now he has time for me). He was acting like he was on a fishing trip, and I told him, the superintendent has the message and she's on her way there. I suggest you get the message from her and hung up. I haven't heard a word from the school since.

Later the Office Coordinator from the MD's office called and said we reviewed the matter concerning the faxing of that document to your son's school and find that we were totally in the wrong and we are very sorry.

I said if this was supposed to be good enough. What about this MD? Is she just supposed to get a slap on the wrist and it's okay to violate my son's civil rights? She said, "no, what would you like to see done with her?"

I said first I wanted an apology from the doctor. I want that doctor to sit down and watch the Lyme CD I just purchased featuring Dr.'s B and B so she can get educated about the disease for the sake of all her patients. And I want posters about Lyme Disease in her waiting area.

I told them that I had already contacted an attorney and had a lot of things to think about. (Which I really did!). "I don't know what I want to do right now. I'm raising my voice with you and I'm terribly upset and I don't want to talk about it anymore right now."

She said the doctor was right there if I would hold just for a minute. I agreed to hold but they took all day so I just hung up. A few minutes later the phone rang and it was the MD on the phone. She said she was very sorry for the error and she really wanted to make it up to me.

I told her how she made me feel at Ryan's appointment when I tried to get her to test him further. I told her that's why we left her practice and went to MO. And that she had just made an utter fool of me at my son's school, and God help her if she interfered with his ability to get a special education plan for his disease. I said the real bummer was that Ryan really liked her and wanted her to be his doctor.

She almost cried and said she hadn't realized she had been so unapproachable when I had asked for help. She said that she felt terrible for what she had put us through. She asked how can she fix it. I asked if she would watch the CD I bought to educate doctors. She agreed. She also agreed to be the Indiana MD to monitor Ryan and vouch for his illness on his school record to get his IEP in the works.

When she hung up she said, "now I want a longer appointment okay?"

I told her, "you can take all the time with me and my son that you need."

Getting something done about Lyme Disease or any of it's multitude of complications is no small feat. Getting anything done quickly is a miracle.

Chapter XIV

Marjorie Tietjen's Thoughts

One signer of the Declaration of Independence (Dr. Benjamin Rush), who was also George Washington's physician, predicted the following. "Unless we put medical freedom into The Constitution, the time will come when medicine will organize into an undercover dictatorship."

As a chronic Lyme patient, I have become very aware of the almost total control that the pharmaceutical companies, the insurance industry and government agencies already have over our healthcare decisions. Most of us can no longer freely choose the doctors we want treating us. Doctors who are thinking for themselves and who are prescribing preventative or curative treatments, instead of only symptomatic treatments, are being ostracized and persecuted. Hundreds of thousands of sick, disabled and dying people are intentionally being denied proper testing, diagnoses and treatment. Many feel that this is due to the greed of the pharmaceutical companies and perhaps the depopulation goals of the bureaucratic elite. The later isn't such a far-fetched idea.

Henry Kissenger himself, in his National Security Memorandum, advised the President that there were 13 countries in Africa which were growing much too rapidly, were threatening the availability of certain resources, and that we needed to either decrease the birth rate or increase the death rate. Not too long after this proposal, the World health Organization visited these countries with free smallpox vaccines. Several years later 60% of the people, who received these shots, presented with the AIDS virus. A similar scenario took place in NYC. Hepatitis B vaccines were given out free to promiscuous gay men. Soon after, 60% of this population also came down with AIDS.

People in a democratic society should have the freedom to purchase any type of natural or synthetic remedy, hire the doctor of their choice, and be able to make the final decision as to what tests they receive and which labs will do their testing. All this should take place without government interference. Most adults are totally capable of managing their healthcare decisions without the government dictating and controlling the most basic and intimate issues of their lives. Doctors who write our prescriptions are managed by corporations and government agencies, which really do not have our best interests at heart. Therefore, I feel that certain prescription and other medical laws need to be revised or perhaps need to be done away with completely. We would still need physicians to advise and direct us but the ultimate decision as to what we put in our bodies, should be made by the individual. This is one of the most basic of freedoms. We have been conditioned to accept the government in the role of parent, protector and babysitter. The more we allow the government (which is essentially a conglomeration of corporations) to make our decisions for us, the more rights we lose. It is all made to seem as though certain controlling laws are solely for our benefit and protection.

Lyme Disease, its testing, diagnoses and treatment, is a perfect example of total deception and intentional misdiagnoses. Just to give you an idea of the magnitude of this travesty, I will list a few of the many disease labels which have been assigned to patients, many of whom have eventually been tested and found positive for Borrelia burgdorferi, the causative agent of Lyme disease. Most of these patients improve with antibiotics, along with natural treatments, and are able to arrest their degenerative disease process. Some of these labels are: Arrhythmia, Arthralgias, Arthritis, ADD, Autoimmune Diseases, Chronic Fatigue Syndrome, Fibromyalgia, Depression, Multiple Sclerosis, Parkinson's, Sleeping Disorders, Alzheimer's, ALS, Irritable Bowel Syndrome, Scleroderma, Peripheral Neuropathy, Lupus.....and the list goes on. I suggest that people conduct searches on the Internet....Pubmed, or just a general search, which would include their specific disease name and or symptom(s), along with "Lyme Disease". I think you may be very surprised at what you find.

Many of these so-called separate diseases have no known definitive tests, causes or cures. Labels are just handed out according to symptoms and the type of specialist you may be seeing at the time of diagnoses. In fact, most chronically ill patients receive many different diagnoses from varied specialists. Required characteristics or markers, for all these conditions, must not be very specific. As I mentioned in a previous article, this confusion prevents proper treatment and covers up the fact that Lyme disease is not only epidemic in our society, but also pandemic.

Treatment rests on the premise of correct testing and diagnoses. If testing is inaccurate then diagnoses and treatment will be invalid. Patients will only receive symptomatic treatments, which often cause additional health problems, and then require more drugs. This obviously benefits the pharmaceutical companies.

Lyme Disease, its testing, diagnoses and treatment, is an extremely controversial subject. Intelligent and open-minded people are questioning why this should be so. The medical community already has an educational model to go by. Syphilis is a spirochete, is a close cousin of the Bb spirochete and behaves in a very similar way. Syphilis is pleomorphic (changes form), is known to be congenitally transmitted, sexually transmitted and it sometimes requires open-ended antibiotic treatment, just as the Bb spirochete does. Why then are not these aspects being vigorously investigated, concerning Bb? Often one hears the excuse that the medical community is stodgy and slow to accept change. This may be partially true of the lower levels of the general medical community. Most doctors rely on the idea that what they learn in medical school and read in the peer reviewed medical journals, is all truth, based on sound medical research and impartially presented. Unfortunately this is Pollyanna wishful thinking. The upper echelon of the NIH, CDC and other government agencies, which play a large role in educating our doctors, many times, have agendas other than what they would have us believe. As I mentioned before, these organizations don't always have our best interests at heart. Several government institutions have patents on microbes, which many of us are infected with. They know what segments of the population are infected with these microbes but they fail to educate the Red Cross, doctors, health departments or the public as to what diseases have these organisms present or as to the successful treatments available.

If patients who are cognitively impaired, due to Neuroborreliosis, can figure out what appears to be happening, then I'm sure that the highly educated researchers and administrators at the CDC, NIH, among others must also have a clue as to the real magnitude of this health crisis and perhaps the real reason behind it.

Researchers and doctors have been taught that Bb is an ancient microbe and that it is just now being recognized for the problem that it is. Considering the fact that most doctors do not recognize or "believe in" the symptom complex presented by Bb infection, leads one to conclude, that if indeed this organism has been around for thousands of years, there must be something new and perhaps more pathogenic, involving current strains. Certain microbiologists agree there is something unusual about Bb and that what we are experiencing is extremely hardy, pathogenic, and tenacious and may involve more organ systems than the historical variety of the Lyme spirochete. It is suspected that the current strain(s) may be genetically modified. One prominent microbiologist said to me "This bug is just too damn smart!"

It is a known fact that mosquitoes have been genetically engineered to become more efficient vectors for certain diseases. West Nile Virus may be one of these diseases that have had some help from scientists. Ades Japonicus, an experimental strain of mosquito, is said to be one of the most efficient vectors of West Nile Virus. Therefore, it doesn't seem beyond the imagination that ticks may have been manipulated in a similar fashion.

Bb, the causative agent of Lyme disease is pleomorphic. This means that it can mutate into several different forms and as a result, is able to evade the immune system, antibiotics and consequently can make testing very difficult. It can go into hiding and lie dormant for varied periods of time. The medical community recognizes the problem of pleomorphism and the resultant difficulty with testing. Why then do they take the stand that if you test negative, with current testing, that you simply don't have Lyme?

Millions and millions of dollars are collected each year for charities involving all these so-called separate diseases. Supposedly research is looking for causes and cures for all these "unrelated" diseases. Where are all these causes and cures? Where are any of them? All I am noticing are more and more emerging conditions with new labels and only symptomatic treatments. I personally know several people who were misdiagnosed with Multiple Sclerosis. A good friend and now a member of our Lyme disease support group, was misdiagnosed with M.S. for 10 years. During these 10 years she lost a very young child to what she now believes was congenital Lyme disease. She was treated with chemotherapy drugs and other M.S drugs, but only continued to decline. She was finally treated for Lyme with long-term antibiotics and has regained many of her functions. She recently acquired her old hospital records, which stated that 10 years ago her spinal fluid and blood had tested positive for Lyme. The records state that the same blood was supposedly retested and found to be negative. She was then handed the label of M.S. She was never told that she ever tested positive for Lyme. My friend of course was shocked. She encouraged others who were diagnosed with M.S to be tested for Lyme. Several other

M.S patients, that she knows, have now tested positive for Lyme and are slowly improving on antibiotics. My friend is a very caring person and naturally wanted to share these findings with the Multiple Sclerosis Society. At first, those she called seemed interested and wanted her to come speak at a conference. Evidently when this information traveled to those with influence, she was told that she couldn't come and share her story. I have also been told by a reliable source that an M.S. organization was instrumental in shutting down the work of a very prominent microbiologist who was finding Lyme spirochetes in many Multiple Sclerosis patients. Yale, which is one of the main forces behind the non-treatment of Chronic Lyme patients, has been diagnosing an unusual amount of M.S in those with neurological problems. Other doctors in the area.... especially those who specialize in pain treatment, are questioning the huge number of patients, diagnosed by Yale, with M.S.

I believe the time has come to decentralize our healthcare. This may mean chaos for a while but I feel the process is inevitable. We need to become more involved on a personal level with researchers and others who are involved with the health and well-being of our nation and the world. I feel this is the only way to discern their integrity and true motives. Instead of pouring all our hard earned money into the huge conglomerate charities, where we have little control or knowledge as to where our money goes, it would seem much more productive and assuring to support the private researchers of our choice.

Our health is one of our greatest treasures. At this critical time in human history, we need to educate ourselves, investigate, trust our intuitions, and work together for positive change.

Most Lyme tests available, are looking for antibodies, our body's reaction to the Lyme spirochete. As I mentioned before, the Lyme spirochete is very adept at evading our immune system by changing its forms and therefore, testing that relies on detection of antibodies, is very unreliable.

I recently discovered information on a fairly new test, which looks for the actual cell wall deficient form of Bb. It locates the actual germ and therefore is very accurate. It is called the Bowen Q-RiBb test, developed by Dr. JoAnne Whitaker and Eleanor Fort. These researchers are finding this organism in a very large segment of the population. I have spoken with Dr. Whitaker several times and was very impressed by her integrity and genuine sincere interest in bringing out the pandemic nature of this disease. She has witnessed so many people being misdiagnosed with other disease labels, such as, M.S, FM, ALS, CFS, etc. It is an unimaginable situation that so many people are falsely diagnosed and as a result, do not receive proper treatment. People are dying because of these misdiagnoses.

Lida Mattman, who is a microbiologist and the author of "Stealth Pathogens", has studied spirochetes for fifty years. She believes that touching can spread Lyme disease. The spirochete is found in tears, which means that it can contaminate the hands and anything they touch. Scientists are finding that the Lyme spirochete is very hardy and can remain viable for long periods of time. Could this possibly be a mode of transmission for Bb within families? Often entire families are ill. One member may be diagnosed with Lyme, another may be diagnosed with ALS, Parkinson's, Alzheimer's, ADD, Fibromyalgia, etc. More and more patients with these labels are testing positive for Lyme, mycoplasma and other tick-borne co-infections. When treated with proper antibiotics, for a sufficient length of time (often several years is needed), a large percentage are improving. What is needed, of course, is accurate testing and more clinical diagnoses. This means tests are used as an adjunct to clinical diagnoses and not as the main determining factor. The main criteria for diagnoses and treatment should be based on the patient's history and symptoms. However , it appears that doctors have come to rely so much on test results that they can't seem to give a clinical diagnoses without a test to back it up. Or perhaps it is the pressure of malpractice or "management" by the corporations that has shaken their confidence. In any case, this is a great disservice to the patient who is seeking diagnoses and treatment.

Sandi Lanford, a Lyme advocate, states the following

facts concerning the Bowen Test. "Positive Bowen Q-RiBb tests have been challenged but no other test has been able to prove these results to be incorrect. There have been no false positives, for when patients are treated, based on the Bowen results; the patients have shown remarkable improvement in their symptoms. It is also difficult to dismiss the accuracy of Dr. Whitaker's Q-RiBb test, as she has an impressive background in the development of fluorescent assays, evident in numerous published research studies. The results of the original Bowen Q-RiBb were duplicated by Lida Mattman's lab in Michigan. Dr. Mattman was nominated for the Nobel Prize in 1998 for her work on Stealth Pathogens. She is a very highly respected microbiologist. On 316 same draw blood samples, 316 cultured specimens grew out the organism Bb and the Q-RiBb test was positive for all 316. The culture method is the Gold Standard for making a definitive diagnoses of an infectious disease. This statement means that out of 316 blood samples drawn for this particular test, the Bowen lab blood samples came up 100% positive for Bb. The Mattman controls, from the same blood samples, were also 100% positive. The Mattman controls duplicated the Bowen Q-RiBb results."

The Bowen Lab is a research lab and depends on grants, donations and profits from testing, in order to stay in operation and conduct more research. It is my opinion that if this test is more widely used, the results may blow the lid off the Lyme pandemic cover-up.

It is very important here to stress that Lyme is not just a tick-borne disease. Mosquitoes have been found to be loaded with this organism. It has also been found in mites, fleas, well water, African dust, tears, semen and breast milk.

Lyme support groups are reporting that those who received labels such as MS, ALS,CFS,FM, etc, were tested with the Q-RiBb test, found to be positive for Lyme, and then treated, are improving. These results only confirm my long held suspicion that Bb and other microbes, such as mycoplasma, are running rampant through our society. It appears that this situation is being allowed to occur. It is fairly obvious that everything possible is being done to thwart proper testing, diagnoses and curative treatment.

The Michigan State Attorney's Office recently told Dr. Mattman to stop helping doctors diagnose Lyme Disease with her testing, and was threatened with time in jail or a fine of $5,000.00 a day. Dr. Mattman says that it is getting more and more difficult to find human negative controls in the U.S. to supply blood free of Borrelia. It appears that the government and certain "charity" organizations, don't want the public to become aware of this information. Recently state police arrived at her lab with handcuffs and tried to find evidence that she was still conducting this work. Fortunately, they didn't find what they were looking for. However, despite lack of evidence, Dr. Mattman has had to discontinue her very valuable work and leave her lab.

This isn't about promoting a certain lab for financial gain. I really believe that the future of our country may hinge on discovering what the Bowen Lab test results are telling us. Our country is becoming more and more disabled and most people don't even realize it. We are told so often that we are the healthiest nation in the world that we actually believe it. Most people I know are not healthy. Everyone, even the young, seems to have some sort of condition. Many people have several overlapping conditions. This is NOT normal!

Is there a common cause?

I think we better find out before it is too late.

For more information on the Bowen Test, please visit www.bowen.org

CHAPTER XV

War With No Peace

Tim's Story

When I met Sue, she was the healthiest and most vivacious person I had ever met. When people spoke about her, descriptive words like "go-getter", "big heart", and "caring" were often heard. Best of all, she loved me in spite of my shortcomings. She had a way of finding the good in most everyone and the humorous side of any uncomfortable situation. She worked hard and volunteered for every worthwhile organization. I knew when I saw a good woman and married her.

Shortly after we were married, the military kept me even busier, but Sue rarely complained. She filled in when I was not around for chores. She even took a job at the radio station I worked for part time. It wasn't because she had aspirations of becoming a disc jockey. In fact, going live made her feel sick at her stomach. No, she did it to save my ass. My military career would keep me away for up to thirty days at a time and the radio station needed someone to fill my slot. Sue learned my position and held it for me by working my hours when I was away. Sue excelled in the radio world and was soon working three times more than I was and even wrote news clips for the morning show. She was like that. Whatever task she took on, she put her heart and soul into it.

The Lyme Disease was not what we expected to hear when she went in to see the doctor for the flu. From that day on, things were never the same. Sue was always so tired even though she pushed herself to limits no one could see. She kept telling me that she would beat this disease since she was always so healthy. Instead, I have watched her deteriorate day by day.

Sue is strong willed and had a love for life. She found so much joy in getting outdoors, drinking in the sunshine and breathing the fresh air. No, she's terrified of grassy areas and forget camping. She knows that she can be reinfected and said that nothing is worth that happening. She now stays indoors and surfs the net for Lyme Disease information. It will come in handy should she ever be fortunate enough to find a physician ever willing to read and follow protocol. As it is right now, there are none here and Sue cannot travel. She has learned that just because a doctor may be a specialist, it does not mean they are a good physician.

Sue also plans on changing the world where Lyme Disease is concerned. She is, when she is able, working on changing how each state reports the disease on their websites. She is also trying to get legislation passed so that this state can afford to get some doctors here that will not be afraid to clinically diagnose and treat this disease. It's a long haul...like the life of a Lyme Disease victim.

In the meantime, she is trying to clear up this mess with the military. She has taken over writing to the DOD and all concerned. She was the one who took to writing the President and Secretary of The Army. She knows and works the chain of command better than any soldier in the U.S. Army. They give her the same runaround that they have given me, but Sue's determination is stronger than mine. I have spent over twenty years dealing with the military and when they denied me my right to be here for Sue, I washed my hands of them. That was no way to treat a soldier who had gone to the Gulf, taken their injections without objections, and followed orders to the letter without a complaint. And, that was no way to treat a respected military wife when she was in need of life saving measures.

I had heard of Lyme Disease when I was stationed at Ft. Riley, Kansas. But didn't really know what it was. I never received a card, saw a poster, but there was a briefing about protecting yourself out on maneuvers. Watching Sue suffer with this disease, I now know that the word should be at every medical facility, even the military facilities. I know that it was not a common word or publicized at Ft. Sill, Oklahoma. Sue would have taken precautions if she had heard about it being a possibility there. No one ever heard of it at Ft. Sill. In fact, I recall one of the doctors saying that they were on the border as far as the tick map went. But, they could not say that they knew that any Lyme Disease cases were being reported.

The first thing I noticed was Sue's bull-eyes rashes on her left arm. That was so long ago, but I recall there were three and they reappeared when she had a high fever one weekend. What symptoms stand out now are the severe pain, constant fatigue, and the chills and hot spells she gets. This has been difficult to watch and not being able to do anything about it. So when my chance came up to save Sue's life by being here for her, I grabbed it. I did it legally, but the South Korean command refused to honor the orders I held in my hand from PERSCOM. I did what I had to do to save my wife's life.

A family member of a Lyme Disease patient can only be supportive. If that's all anyone learns, it's enough. The doctors that Sue has seen are no supportive. The other family members so not seem to understand what is happening to Sue. The community where she spent so much of her time helping didn't get it. And her friends have all forsaken her. Sue doesn't cry much, but I have seen her shed many tears over this disease. It has cost her everything and no one seems willing to help her get well. If I were a doctor, I would sure pay attention to the complaints of a Lyme Disease patient. The Lymer (as Sue calls herself) knows more than most of the doctors out there. They study the disease, live with the symptoms and suffer each day with embarrassment from not being who they once were.

Sue has trouble speaking most days. She used to have a large vocabulary, not she's lucky to find a simple word to express her thought or idea. She can no longer drive or do the shopping. That now falls on me. What irks me is that no one seems to give a damn. Not the doctors, the government, or the military. This disease is worse than SARS, but that's all we heard about when a few cases broke out. Last year, Sue was given less than five years left to live. The reports say that Lyme Disease doesn't kill!

This disease has an effect on everyone. Sue's mom and dad aren't doing well medically speaking. They can't make the trip to see Sue and she can't make the trip anymore to visit with them. That's all the family Sue has, besides my folks. And, my folks aren't in the best of shape either. When I was asked why I hadn't moved Sue closer to family, the military didn't want to hear that no one was able to help Sue if she needed anything. They didn't want to understand anything except some soldier in South Korea may need a driver's permit and I was expected to be there to hand it to them. Even when they knew I was not supposed to be in Area I, they brushed this under the carpet. They knew it was against regulations, but that I would probably never say anything because I was a soldier. The military breaks and bends rules all the time, but very few soldiers ever say anything. If one does, he or she pays for it tenfold.

If there were things that could be in place in the military to prevent someone from ever having to endure what Sue and I have gone through, that would be wonderful. There should be compassionate reassignments allowed for Lyme Disease. After hearing about Michael Carroll's book about Lab 257 on Plum Island, I would think that the military would be more understanding about this disease.

We have lost everything because of the disease and the way the military is handling it. Even though we have Congressionals and active military investigations ongoing, these have not reinstated my military pay, my retirement or carried on our privileges. We have been reduced to borrowing money, living on peanut butter and jelly, and layering clothes to save on heating costs. We cannot afford anything and that includes Sue's medications. She has now connected with other Lyme Disease patients to get her Doxycycline. Instead of the Motrin that helps her with the pain, she is reduced to taking whatever she can to get through the days.

It breaks my heart to see suffer and degraded. It makes me angry that the twenty years I served this country seems to mean nothing. I was only a eight months from retirement. I was under legitimate orders to be here with Sue. I was doing what was morally and legally right. When I filed a complaint against the South Korean command, it seems that anyone who could do anything about it turned their attention away from the regulations. This actually didn't surprise us, but I can't imagine that the investigations have gone on almost a year and no one has any results, answers or has deemed this necessary to straighten out.

Sue writes and three months later, she gets a letter from DOD stating that they need more time. The last letter, dated December 16, 2003, was from a Lt. Colonel stating that the agencies he has been waiting on to respond has not done so. Could it be the South Korean command he is waiting on and they have nothing to back up what they did? How long before anyone realizes this? Are they waiting for command to change to a new commander and brush this all under a rug? Sue sent the Lt. Colonel over four hundred documents to back up the claim that this was all illegally done and who was responsible. This was never acknowledged, but was signed for.

Even though we have lost everything we worked for all of our lives, have been reduced to below poverty level, and have had to wonder where Sue would get the medications that keep her alive with this disease....we are still here. Sue fights for her life and we wait in purgatory while the military ignores what they have done to send us here.

Next time you see a soldier in uniform, please think of this soldier who served his country with pride. I am no longer proud to have been part of such a corrupt bunch of green suits or that I wasted those years believing what the military taught me. It isn't true that they take care of their own. They are too busy taking care of other countries to worry about any soldier trying to save his wife from dying.

When I recall the seven Army values, I wonder when the same soldiers who denied me a compassionate reassignment will ever live up to the same set I was to live by.

Loyalty
Bear true faith and allegiance to the U.S. constitution, the Army, and other soldiers.
Be loyal to the nation and its heritage.
Duty
Fulfill your obligations.

Accept responsibility for your own actions and those entrusted to your care.

Find opportunities to improve oneself for the good of the group.

Respect

Rely upon the golden rule.

How we consider others reflects upon each of us, both personally and as a professional organization.

Selfless Service

Put the welfare of the nation, the Army, and your subordinates before your own.

Selfless service leads to organizational teamwork and encompasses discipline, self-control and faith in the system.

Honor

Live up to all the Army values

Integrity

Do what is right, legally and morally.

Be willing to do what is right even when no one is looking.

It is our "moral compass" an inner voice.

Personal Courage

Our ability to face fear, danger, or adversity, both physical and moral courage

Sue has constitutional rights and I, as a soldier, should protect her rights. So, I was being "loyal". I fulfilled my obligations and was accepting responsibility for my wife's care. This is "duty". "Do unto others as you would have them do unto you" is the golden rule. I couldn't have been more considerate to the military or my wife. I was in possession of valid orders and I was making sure my wife would receive the care she desperately needed to live. I certainly believe this was "respect".

I put the Army first over twenty years and would have been able to juggle both, my career and Sue's care, if I had been granted a compassionate reassignment. But, I was never given the opportunity. Instead, the South Korean command illegally listed me as AWOL and ruined my career. I was a selfless servant over twenty years. And, until this happened, was proud of being part of the U.S. Army. I was also doing what was morally and legally right. It was the U.S. Army that failed. I have integrity. Sue and I, both, have more courage than we know what to do with. We have been forced to face the entire U.S. Army, the White House, among others. Even though they can't get their act together enough to straighten this mess they have created out, we still face them with courage. That's been the easy part. We have documentation to prove what they did was illegal, immoral, and appalling. The DOD say they cannot get their agencies to give them reports or documentation that will complete their investigation? What values do all these people live by? It surely can't be the seven I have practiced for over twenty years.

Chapter XVII

Humor and Lyme Disease

Once I was past the depression of the disease, AWOL status, losing everything, and moving to this place that I never expected to be, I found humor again. In the past, I had been the one to laugh at myself for mistakes and shortcomings, help others to find the "up side" of things, and cheer up a sad situation. Now, if you will, enjoy how I see things now through these Lymer eyes. Living in what I now to refer to as The Hole.

I have described moving to the Midwest, but I never told you how we live or what I see when I look out of the front windows. No, it's not the boarded up windows of the storefronts across the street or the one skinny tree barely surviving on the corner. It's not the Hilton or even a nice town. But the apartment and the residents are what keep me giggling. The quarters are a hoot and the folks are unaware of their eccentricities. Free entertainment is always something I can handle, even before we ended up broke.

The apartment is a one-bedroom, smaller than small, used-to-be dress shop. This means that we have two show room windows to provide an almost unlimited view of the settlement here and the comings and goings of most of the people.

Of course the apartment is on the first of two floors; Lymers have problems negotiating steps. Walking through the front door, you are immersed in a blue-green sea, okay a puddle, of worn carpet, dark beige walls topped with a mauve-blue-brown flower border from the 40's. I warned you that it wasn't the Hilton. Watch your step as you come though, there are weak boards in front of the front door (shower, too). You're just liable to fall through to the basement.

Standing in the middle of the room, you can make a complete circle and see the hub of our little asylum. It's an 18 x 15 foot room and in it we have a living-kitchen-dining-room and office space. Behind the loveseat is our storage area just as under the end table serves the same purpose. We take full advantage of every nook and cranny here. This is where we have suitcases packed with summer clothes and our camping equipment. We use under the bed storage, but we have long forgotten what is under there.

Through the doorway (no door), you'll find the miniature bedroom. And, through another door to the left, you find yourself in a bathroom. Sounds pretty simple and straightforward, but nothing in my life is ever uncomplicated since Lyme Disease. The commode is partially blocked by a heating duct so doing what comes naturally has to be done in a most unnatural position. It can only be described as a lifting-shifting-posing-balancing-juggling kind of act. The shower is not for the faint of heart or claustrophobic. It's so small and dark that one can imagine what a coffin is like. And forget a hot shower. I believe that the water heater is in proportion to the apartment, tiny.

In the living area, there's not a whole lot of room for furniture. When we moved in, we had nothing but two camp chairs and a cooler, so it felt like a football field. Okay, a sandbox. We have come a long way, borrowing, garage sales and dumpster diving. It's amazing what you can do with the used, abused, and worn out.

The first thing we borrowed was a bed and we were thrilled when my daughter-in-law's folks threw in a set of sheets. We went to Goodwill and bought a desk, a lamp, and two bowls for food. A barn auction was the home to our loveseat, but it was only $10.00 and with a cover, not a bad place to sit. Personally, I still prefer the camp chairs.

We borrowed a dinette set and two cheap bookcases. I suppose that the dinette was cheap too since two of the chairs have broken and the last fall nearly killed me. Everything in the hole has to have a dual use. The dinette doubles as a workstation for projects, a laundry table, and a place to keep the toaster. The bookcases serve as our dressers, with laundry baskets holding our clothes. Hey! We each have our own and it's working out nicely. In the bottom of the bookcase, we can store some shoes and a couple of books.

In the kitchen area, the counter tilts two inches towards the center of the room. The stovetop is part of the counter and it makes cooking a tricky task. For example, eggs seem to want to run towards one side of the skillet, as does the cooking oil. The food cooks unevenly, but a knife under one side of the pan evens it all out.

Washing dishes is always an experience here and we have yet to get this down to an art. Of course it could be due to the sink's size, a twelve-inch square. Water splashes everywhere and nothing but a glass and cup fit in it together at one time. We noticed that the cabinet underneath was always wet, but a thick line of silicone along the cook top edge fixed this right up.

We were told that this dump was insulated. However, after being here over ten months, we have found little proof of this claim. Unless the landlords were possibly referring to the carpet that runs up the wall about four inches as insulation, there seems to be none. We know that it's hopelessly cold in the winter and damned hot in the summer. But, it's our "home zany home".

The queen-size bed literally fills the bedroom. Tim has learned to be a contortionist in order to change the bedclothes. This is sure to count as exercise! This, I suppose, is when I am thankful that I hurt too much to even attempt the changing of the sheets. Getting the constant everyday layers of dust off the walls and curtains from a dumpster diving expedition is the real exercise we get here. Someone holds the vacuum cleaner up (we found that sitting it on top of the bed just causes the rotating brushes to snag the blankets and chews holes), and the other person stands shoeless on the bed, guiding the vacuum hose to suck up the dust bunnies. It's quite a workout.

We now do our laundry in the apartment as opposed to taking it to a neighbor's. A small used washer (knob missing, but pliers work) that hooks up to the tiny sink and we're in business. However, I was used to the regular sized washers and it took me almost two months before I discovered the right ratio of detergent and water. In the meantime, Tim said we were exfoliating after our showers (no room for a bathtub here). The towels were always stiff as boards. Doing laundry could be viewed as a poor woman's spa. The washer vibrates so much that I have to lay across it to keep it from unplugging itself (a reducing machine), I walk back and forth hundreds of times loading and unloading each piece (a treadmill), the towels are rough (exfoliating, I hear costs a lot at a real spa), and on a hot day, it all feels like a sauna.

To dry our laundry during the summer months, I started out with 5-50 cord (green rope used for parachutes) strung from side to side under the awning over our front door. This idea didn't work out as the clothes dragged the ground. I next came up with the "clothes hangar-clothes pin" drying method, which wasn't such a bad idea. I would hang, for example, a towel on the clothes hangar with two clothes pins and hook the hangar on slits under the awning. This served a couple of purposes; no one could get through the soldiers of clothes for a visit and it provided entertainment for the neighborhood. I was soon regarded as the Chinese Laundry Lady. But one afternoon it would take on a whole new connotation. A woman from down the block, better known as drug block C, came by and was pawing through our laundry. When I came out, she asked how much my nightshirt was! She said that she imagined that we were having a garage sale, but was a little miffed that nothing had been priced.

We have some colorful town folk here. There's Cowboy Bob, Sally the Slumlord, and high-water Harry. These three are regulars at the nucleus of this universe, the U.S. Post Office.

It's a small, one room building. One side is lined with mailboxes (key rental is $2.00 for life-God, please don't let us have to stay here that long) and the other side is a counter with one lonely employee who knows it all. Everyone must visit the heart of the town in order to receive mail. There is no such thing as delivery inside the "city limits".

Cowboy Bob is a tall, gangly man, I guess to be in his sixties. His beard is gray, so I assume the hair on his head is, too. But, I couldn't swear to this. Bob has a bargain basement dirty, straw cowboy hat on during any season and in all weather conditions. Same applies for the waist-length soiled coat he sports. His companion is a curled wooden staff that measures at least seven feet. He never speaks to anyone, but will tip his hat to a lady as he passes. Now I know where chivalry went!

Sally is one of the landlords on Block C of this tiny community. She is in her seventies, but dresses like a twenty year-old hooker. Her skirts are tight and short and she is definitely into leopard prints. Sally's hair is dyed a rust color and her lipstick is bright ruby red (this is to match her rouge). Sally stopped a couple of times as I sat outside and her story was less than charming. Seems that her tenants were unhappy about their commode not working. She couldn't figure out why they had been complaining for the last four months...evidently they had found a place to "go" in all that time. Never a dull moment here!

High-water Harry is a bachelor and cream of the crop here. He weighs in at about fifty pounds dripping wet and stands no more than five feet tall. No matter what the weather, Harry has an imitation black leather jacket on, a white dress shirt and jeans that show creases from being pressed. From the shins down is where the dilemma lies. The hem of his jeans has never been introduced to his brown shoes or white socks. I can't imagine why Harry is still single. He seems like such a lovely man.

I just have to tell you about the biggest attractions here...parades! The first one was the talk of the town long before it ever took place. We were told that it would be on the 4th of July, to set up our lawn chairs, and get ready for an "good time". I made iced tea, dug through a suitcase for our sun-visors and moved our chairs right out in front of our apartment (we were assured that the parade route came right past us, weren't WE the lucky couple). Tim was working nights and had only had a couple of hours rest when I roused him for the event. He rubbed his eyes and eventually found his way to a camp chair. I knew he was humoring me and would rather be chewing glass than waiting for a parade. But, there we were, along with every other resident in town.

The police cruiser sirens announced the start of the procession. Someone whispered that the cop (who was our one and only and also served as the preacher here) had actually washed the squad car. Next was the one and only fire truck with kids waving from the top. Following behind the big red truck was a convertible filled with more waving children and the finale, a garden tractor. The operator was clad in a checkered shirt and straw hat, but this was the only embellishment to the entire parade. Then, it was over! Needless to say, Tim was less than thrilled that I had gotten him up from a much deserved sleep for this. But, it only lasted ten minutes. No real harm done.

We didn't see the last parade coming. We were watching television and heard sirens blaring from what seemed like all directions. We rushed outside just in time to see the familiar police car and fire truck passing by. The local baseball team had won and this was the celebration. We would have prepared iced tea and arranged our camp chairs...but there just wasn't time!

Lolly and Dolly have an interesting line of business, obesity. Really! They are an unmarried couple who have learned that being overweight is a lucrative diversion from real employment. They get checks from the government for being "fat". Being obese makes them unable to work so therefore, they are entitled to an income. And they are pretty darned proud of this means of income, too. To hear them talk, they wouldn't have it any other way. Their sideline though is garbage picking for resalable items. The chair that was at the curb for trash day somehow ended up in the one of the few businesses left open here, an antique store. But, when they raided the neighbor's trash, they made the foolish mistake of trying to sell the goods door-to-door. One of the doors they knocked on belonged to the neighbor's brother and the item was a broken chainsaw that he had personally set out as refuse. No sale there! But hearing the neighbor's brother tell and retell the story, I would imagine it will soon become a legend.

The water here has so many chemicals in it that it has ruined three coffee pots and caused my doctor to comment on my dry skin (yes, I use lotion, but as far as I know, there's no industrial strength creams out).

Things I have learned include, clothes pins are handy for curtain tie backs, chip clips for bags, note holders, paper clips, and an emergency hair clip. Poor people buying a new vacuum cleaner is equivalent to purchasing a new car. Money is tight and "on sale" doesn't always mean a bargain. One can live without an oven because there are toaster ovens (no one seemed to be able to find room for an oven when they installed the sink here). A butter knife can be used to pry, pound, screw, and level saving room in the drawer for forks and spoons. You CAN get three cups out of a Folger's coffee bag and have it taste just fine. Add water to the half bottle of shampoo or dish soap; it goes further and cleans just the same. Wash cloths do just as well for washing dishes as rags marked, "dish cloths". Glue, brads, and tape can fix almost anything you find in a dumpster. Invest in a good clothes-drying rack for indoor, winter drying. If not, get two rolls of duct tape for repairs and reinforcement. Duct tape can also be used to repair CPAP hoses and to seal cracks around the windows. Rolled towels work just as well as those store-bought draft guards. Cutting up a fallen tree from a storm CAN be a fun event. A couple of interested neighbors who are amused by watching paint dry, a few scattered lawn chairs, and a jug of lemonade...that's the makings of a party here. Painting half the building a dull yellow over grubby beige is NOT an improvement, insulation comes in spray or roll (not at the end of carpet), and noisy neighbors ARE a problem. Bingo winners are supposed to be paid in cash, not pull tabs. There IS more to life than bologna at a function. Canned meat can be good with enough gravy. And lastly, that pipe that sticks out in front of the commode five inches cannot be decorated to look as if it fits in. It makes for a tough time to finish business too. Sitting on a wobbly ring with the necessity to cross your legs is just not natural and could possibly cause long lasting psychological effects (we are still doing research).

We all have gifts. Having Lyme Disease brought out my hidden gift of writing. The military forced me to use it.

Two woman, suffering with Lyme Disease, have found their gifts in art. They have graciously agreed to share some of their talent with you. The spheres can be energizing or relaxing. I have four of Barb's spheres framed and hanging where I need them most, at my desk. The cartoons are fun, surreal and some say what most Lymers feel. Thank you ladies for your contribution.

There is no evidence that supports the theory that life is serious. So at your next Lyme Disease party, try some new games; musical recliners, but note that some Lymers will hear their own music (musical hallucinations); spin the bottle of antibiotics (your choice of doxy or amoxy); pin the Lyme on the tick (you don't have to be blindfolded, but you must wear light colored clothing); 20 questions (this game could take awhile since Lymers forget everything in ten seconds or less); and, Lymer Says (played like Simon Says, but canes and walkers need to be figured in).

Some cute one-liners: Seen it, done it, don't recall it; Thou shall not steal, the government and insurance companies hate competition; Support bacteria, it's not the only culture that the government has; Just when I got a handle on life, it broke; and, a penny saved is an oversight.

Did you ever have one of these days? You put your shoes on and your spouse points out, "you have your shoes on the wrong feet, Dear." You reply, "don't kid me, Buster, I still KNOW my own feet!" Did you ever feel like your life had an outstanding cast on stage, but you could never grasp the plot?

Do you think Lyme Disease research has come to no final conclusion because where we are right now is where the scientists got tired of thinking and just stopped? Is this why the research studies look like surveillance instead of diagnostic trials?

There are some big ole' lies and I am sure we have heard them all, but, I firmly support repeating. Here's the top ten lies...1) I'm from the government and we're here to help you, 2) It's MS, Lupus, (or insert anything you like), because we don't have Lyme Disease here, 3) it's all in your head, 4) you're cured, 5) it's only going to hurt a little while, 6) 30 days of antibiotics is all you need, 7) any doctor can treat Lyme Disease, 8) it's just stress, 9) we are studying Lyme Disease to make things better, 10) the insurance companies/pharmaceuticals/universities are your friends.

For those that don't have this disease, please think before you ask us questions. We may be sick, but the person that we have always been is still in here somewhere. Don't ask what Lyme Disease is. Do your homework. Don't tell us that Cousin Billy-Bob's friend had this and was cured in a week. There is no cure. Don't tell us that we look just fine or be miffed after not seeing us for a month that we are STILL sick. It's not a common cold. Please don't suggest we see a doctor. We probably have seen more doctors than you have fingers or toes. We don't need your sympathy or even complete understanding. We would just like you to treat us as you would want to be treated. We have given up our dignity by just having this disease and its complications. When we are having a Lyme fog, don't tell us that you "just told us" whatever it was you just told us. You wouldn't expect a plane to be able to land in dense fog; don't expect us to always be clear on the landing strip. Just because we are sick, this does not mean that we are immune to unkind people. Be patient with us. We are ALL a work in progress. It's just that our progress is different and may be on a slower pathway than yours. In the end, just be our friend, brother, sister, mother, father, aunt, uncle, or whatever title you held before we became ill. Please include us in whatever we were included in before the disease. But, excuse us if the plans we have made must be canceled. We never know when a bad day will come or what will hurt next or even how fatigued we will feel. We already know we are "no fun anymore". We don't need reminding. It's not that we have changed, but that Lyme Disease has changed our lifestyles. We would like to still be active, volunteering, working or planning a long-term future. It's exhausting enough for us to just get through hours or days with this disease. When we feel badly, just knowing that someone cares enough to bring a little chicken soup or offers to make a trip to the store for us is a gesture that is greatly appreciated. Don't think that our moods are something that can be controlled by us. We sometimes feel angry or blue just because. We don't understand anymore than you do about these frames of mind. We may seem anxious, but we cannot explain it to anyone. It just "is".

When someone figures this disease out and treatment is available that will get us back to "normal", we hope that our family and friends will still be in tact. We have seen so many go through divorce, loss of relationships, and even isolation because of Lyme Disease and the complications it imposes on us. We are not crazy, insane, or idiotic. We are just too ill to help you understand, cope and survive. Underneath it all, we are still the same person you have always known. Help us to remember that by being the same person we have always known.

Compassion, patience, kindness and consideration are key words when dealing with the ill. Life goes on around us and we sometimes feel excluded, accidentally or intentionally. It's not possible at times for us to just get out of the house, exercise, or even make a meal. Even if we DID do it yesterday. We get our medication out to take, remove the lid, and just that quick, we aren't sure if we have taken the pill or not. We have been making that special meatloaf all of our lives. We question ourselves constantly; did I put the eggs in, the special seasoning, or what temperature does it cook at? Did I turn off the stove, the coffee pot, or the water? We appear to be OCD (obsessive compulsive disorder), but know that if we did not have Lyme Disease, we would not have to be questioning ourselves. It's the brain fog and cognitive issues that make us unsure and forgetful. Just imagine yourself in a thick cloud, not being able to tell up from down.

I have gotten lost, but it's always a new adventure. When the doctor heard about this, he asked that I give up driving. I thought that he was concerned with my welfare until I overheard him explain to his nurse about my situation. It seems that the doctor was worried that he would be on the same road as me. I would have waved, promise!

My eyesight is failing, but the optician claimed that I could never wear one set of glasses. The top and bottom seem to be the problem, but the middle was fine. Now, if I could figure out where the middle of my eyesight is, I wouldn't need glasses at all.

My fingers and neck tingle and I have a stabbing pain in my big toe at night. I associate this with the way I used to feel after I tried to find my way to the bathroom in the dark. Tingly when I bumped into a door frame and the stabbing pain when my foot found the chair leg.

Speech is a big problem for most Lymers. I have no trouble at all these days. In fact, I could probably write a new dictionary of the words I have invented trying to convey a thought. One or two have caught on, but we have lost their meanings. It's just fillers and when one Lymer is talking with another, we just seem to know what the words mean. If I could remember how to spell, we'd all be in business.

I have noticed that I have developed sensitivities. This includes odors, chemicals, lights, weather, and noises. Popcorn is the one thing that can make me queasy before the first kernel is heated. I can't tolerate colognes and cleaning fluids break me out and tends to make my hands swell three times their size. Intense lights give me a headache. I feel like Goldie Locks with regards to the weather...too hot, too cold, just right. Noises have to be the worse. My husband sits across the room to enjoy his popcorn, watching the wrestlers, all the lights turned on, and his aftershave screaming that it's too much...I don my headphones and sunglasses, slip a peppermint in my mouth for nausea, wrap up in a blanket and sit back to enjoy our little institution of harmony. Togetherness!

Each morning, I have a runny nose, can't seem to move my joints and am dizzy until my piece of toast. Throw in some light twitching and fatigue no matter how many hours of sleep you get. No wonder Tim makes coffee and leaves me alone for the first hour after I drag my body out of bed. It's a wonder we are still married since on top of all this, we gave up sex, kissing, and sharing a soft drink after I was diagnosed with Lyme Disease. This is true love!

Speaking of true love, it was proven twice since Lyme Disease. The first time came within a week after my gallbladder surgery. Tim and I had been on leave before his tour in South Korea. We were shopping at a mall and I suddenly felt exhausted. I waited in the car for Tim to return from purchasing an item. I felt, in the twinkle of an eye, like I had to go to the bathroom. I didn't wait, but barley made it to the end of the car before all hell breaks loose. I got back in the car, saving anyone else the sight of a wall-less outhouse. I was hysterical with laughter by the time finished his shopping, but he did not share my sentiment. However, he rushed me to the nearest gas station so I could clean myself up. He was so sweet and washed the seat without a word. The second time the expression of love came when we were in a restaurant parking lot. I didn't get a warning this time, but I noticed that I was wearing the same yellow shorts and blue shirt. I told Tim that I had figured out why this was happening, but I don't think he bought it.

Lyme Disease victims deal with lots of insomnia. I can't explain this, but just go with the flow of things. It saves time and effort from trying to change what cannot be made different. I can't read much. I get tired of having to start over after a couple of paragraphs because I have forgotten what I read a minute ago. I look at photo albums, but can't attest that these faces belong to my side of the family. I have tried puzzles of all kinds on those nights I can't sleep. Word puzzles of any kind remind me of looking for a needle in a haystack. Lymers are lacking in the concentration and attention department at times, and when I can't sleep, these are my times.

My heart races, my eyes are blurry, and I have gained weight. I herx, suffer from yeast infections, and pains are migrating. When

I get old, I will already be experienced. Those little old ladies in the nursing home will have nothing on me!

My cats remind me that it's treat-time by sitting at my feet and staring at me. They are so good at being little time pieces. As if on queue at 8, noon, and 6, there they are. My friends call me to make me remember that aliens haven't landed yet. It's better than any news program on television. My neighbors make so much noise that I know there are others living their lives as they choose. I will be happy to leave all of this behind, however. I am looking for bigger and better adventures that will turn my giggles into fall down laughter. I am sure it's somewhere warm, cloudy, quiet, and odor free. I have become quite quirky, but in spite of it all, my husband still adores me.

Chapter XVIII

Surviving In Spite of It ALL

So, here we are, in purgatory. That place that we have been sentenced to without being heard. We got here by way of the military and the way they decide the need for a soldier to be compassionately reassigned. We landed on our knees because the military look at Lyme Disease as not a medical necessity or just cause for a reassignment. The complications, even though they can be life threatening, are also no reason for the soldier to be considered for a compassionate reassignment, in the eyes of the military.

We live from hand to mouth, in fear of losing what little we have left, and in agony that this may never end. We never intentionally hurt anyone and do not understand how this all came to be. While I was fighting for my life with the assistance of my husband, the military decided that the surgery to save my life was "elective". While still with days on legal orders, the South Korean command decides to list Tim as AWOL, leaving us without income or insurance. When presented with the facts and documents to support the facts, the Pentagon and White House ignore everything that is proper, but sustain the illegal actions of those under their command.

We gave our life to this country, as many American do on a daily basis. We worked for what we believed was the good of all.

Tim and I are opposed to injustice and when seeing it in the military family, we always considered it an oversight or mistake. Until this happened to us, we never considered that anything the military did to their own was deliberate harm. However, we have come to look at this situation in a different light as the weeks turn into months and the months into years. I ask questions and am given vague responses. I write letters with supporting documents and it appears that they are disregarded. I ask government officials for help, they tell me how appalled they are at this situation, and within a short period of time, they disappear. There seems to be no rhyme or reason to the antics of our government.

Because of Lyme Disease, I got sick and the military decided that this was no grounds for a compassionate reassignment. Now, I have to find out where this disease comes from since it has been hinted that the military created this in a laboratory. If this is the case, then the military was not only wrong in disregarding Tim's legal orders, but I hold them responsible for making me sick enough to get us to the point of even needing a compassionate reassignment in the first place. If they produced this, then they are fully aware of what this disease can do and how ill we become. They must be aware that we are suffering with the disease and complications from the disease. Therefore, it would be understandable that they would realize that a person with Lyme Disease needs assistance for the disease and the complications. Ergo, it would be only common sense thinking that a compassionate reassignment would be the first step in obtaining the medical treatment necessary for the disease and its complications.

But, what if the military didn't want anyone to know that Lyme Disease was produced in their laboratories? What if someone was ill with Lyme Disease and that person embarrassed the military in South Korea? Would this not be a reason they would not want the Lymer to get any help? I know that this was a consideration, as far as I was concerned. You don't treat someone so harshly and then have the bigwigs in Washington ignore that illegal treatment, especially when it's a soldier with a spotless record and a wife who has taught their new wives how to behave as the military suggests. What other explanation could there be?

If the military had made an innocent mistake, they have had over 400 documents sent in support of my claims and almost a year to clear this all up. There would have been no story, no need to approach the media, and certainly no book. However, there has been no advance on the military's part to get anything straightened out.

If the military had been too busy to take care of this situation, that would be understandable. However, again, they have had plenty of opportunities and time to reinstate Tim's good name, his retirement, and all benefits. This has not happened.

I am not angry at the military, as a whole, for their hand in these illegal actions. Our soldiers are the best of the best, but we evidently have a few rotten apples among the crop of wonderful, selfless, heroes. I am certainly disappointed that a select few, in every link of the chain of command, felt the need to humiliate us for revenge.

This ordeal has taught me invaluable lessons and for this I am thankful. I would never have known all the wonderful people that I have met in dealing with this disease. They have supported us when we needed it most and it had nothing to do with what rank my husband wore or what we had accomplished. It did not matter that we were now poor and could not tender anything in return. We learned to accept the type of support that we had always been known for, but had never been in a position to seek.

We have learned humility. When you are inside a dumpster looking for anything useful because you have nothing, it suddenly hits you. This is the bottom and you got here, not because you had done anything inhumane, but because you did the right thing. We have taken each day, one at a time. Somewhere, sometime, the truth will come out. There will be justice, and we can again return to live freely America. As it stands right now, we feel fortunate that we still have dignity in knowing that what was done to us was through no fault of our own.

We have gone through the stages of grief, with Lyme Disease and the military's way of dealing with this disease. Shock, the first step, when we learned that I had this debilitating disease and shock again, when the military revealed that this disease was not important enough to reassign a soldier with compassion. Denial was my middle name for four years after being diagnosed and denial again when the military was not allowing a compassionate reassignment because of the disease (we just felt this was a huge mistake and nothing more). Then, anger hit. This was the toughest of all the steps. It was not easy for us to get angry and especially at the military. They had been revered in our home and lives for forever. And, we got angry at this disease. How could this have happened to me? What had we done to deserve this punishment? We finally worked our way to acceptance. This isn't to mean that we just gave in or gave up. No, it meant much more. We decided to turn all that we had been through into something good, no matter what the cost. I began to throw myself into researching the people and organizations involved with this disease. I joined support groups to learn as well as give support. Tim supports me as he always has done, 110%. It has made us stronger and better to each other.

So, in the end, we may have had to borrow, beg, and rummage through trash, but we have benefited from the experience. Our concentration has been focused on getting the military to right the wrong that they have done. This focus will not alter or be influenced. We have seen the bottom of the barrel and have survived in spite of the iniquity. But, we are entitled to have Tim's name returned to good standing with back pay, his retirement approved, and all benefits reinstated. We have the right to have our belongings returned from South Korea immediately and a final move addressed. This is all that we are asking because it's what we deserve.

Lyme Disease victims look for answers. Daily, I search for solutions, reading everything in connection with this disease. I speak with others and learn what they know. I believe that someone has the answers to my questions and possibly the key to this disease. I have nothing else better to invest my time in than Lyme Disease and its complications (medical and otherwise).

I believe there is a reason that Lyme Disease exists. I know that there is a reason that no one has found a solution or treatment for this disease. Exploring, with these two statements in mind, I will continue to search for the truth, justice, and American way. It is my duty as a Lyme Disease victim, a human being, and an American.

We have been yelled at, held against our will, and humiliated. We have been reduced to poverty and forced to accept the military's feeble explanations as to why they cannot straighten this all out. But, for all that we have endured at the hands of the military, we are still here. They forgot one important ingredient in their actions and that is our will to survive...in spite of it all.

DIAGNOSTIC HINTS AND TREATMENT GUIDELINES FOR LYME AND OTHER TICK BORNE ILLNESSES

JOSEPH J. BURRASCANO JR., M.D.

Fourteenth Edition
November, 2002
Copyright, November, 2002

INTRODUCTION

Welcome to the fourteenth edition of the "Guidelines." With the passage of time, our understanding of tick-borne illness has grown, so new information is presented to help us further refine our management techniques.

"Lyme Disease" is not simply an infection with *Borrelia burgdorferi*, but a complex illness potentially complicated by multiple tick-borne co-infections. In later stages, it also includes a very significant degree of immune suppression. This not only serves to perpetuate the infections, but it is probably responsible for the reactivation of latent infections, such as herpes-type viruses. Many collateral conditions result in those who have been chronically ill so it is not surprising that damage to virtually all bodily systems can result. To fully recover, all of these issues must be addressed in a thorough and systematic manner. No single treatment or medication will result in full recovery of the more ill patient. Only by addressing all these smaller issues and engineering treatments and solutions for all of them will we be able to restore full health to our patients.

Once again, the full spectrum of Lyme Borreliosis will be addressed, from the new bite, through early and late disseminated infections, and certainly to chronic Lyme Disease.

A very important issue is the definition of "Chronic Lyme Disease." Based on my clinical data and the latest published information, I offer the following definition. To be said to have chronic Lyme, these three criteria must be present:

    Illness present for at least one year

    Have persistent major neurologic involvement (such as encephalitis/encephalopathy, meningitis, etc.) or active arthritic manifestations (active synovitis).

    Still have active infection with B. burgdorferi, regardless of prior antibiotic therapy (if any).

It is clear that in the great majority of patients, chronic Lyme is a disease affecting predominantly the nervous system. Thus, careful evaluation often includes neuropsychiatric testing, SPECT and MRI brain scans, CSF analysis when appropriate, regular input from Lyme-aware neurologists and psychiatrists, pain clinics, and occasionally specialists in psychopharmacology.

As an extension of the effect of chronic Lyme Disease on the central nervous system, new information has demonstrated a deleterious effect on the hypothalamic-pituitary axis. Varying degrees of pituitary insufficiency are being seen in these patients, the correction of which has resulted in restoration of energy, stamina and libido, and resolution of persistent hypotension. Unfortunately, not all specialists recognize pituitary insufficiency, partly because of the difficulty in making the laboratory diagnosis. However, the potential benefits of diagnosing and treating this justify the effort needed for full evaluation.

The concept of a "therapeutic alliance" between the caregiver and patient must again be emphasized. This means that the patient has to work with and become part of the medical team, and must take responsibility for complying with the recommendations given, maintaining the best possible health status, reporting promptly any problems or new symptoms, and especially in realizing that despite all our best efforts, success in diagnosis and treatment is never assured. The medical team must make great efforts to listen carefully to the patient and not be too quick to dismiss seemingly bizarre or illogical complaints.

I once again extend my best wishes to the many patients and caregivers who deal with Lyme, and a sincere thank you to my colleagues whose endless contributions have helped me shape my approach to tick borne illnesses. I hope that my new edition proves to be useful. Happy reading!

BACKGROUND INFORMATION
SPIROCHETE LOAD AND IMMUNE SUPPRESSION IN LYME DISEASE

The spirochete load has a direct bearing on the severity of Lyme presentation. Low spirochete loads result in mild or even inapparent infections that can be missed and remain present for years. As spirochete load increases, especially from subsequent tick bites, the morbidity of Lyme increases. Symptoms become apparent and more debilitating the larger the load, and testing for Lyme can become more accurate. Studies have shown that higher loads also begin to clinically impact the immune system, with invasion and killing of B- and T-lymphocytes, including Natural Killer Cells, and inhibition of lymphocyte transformation and mitogenesis. A corollary to the issue of spirochete load is the delicate balance between defense efficacy vs. pathogen strength. In other words, more severe illness also results from weakened defenses, such as from severe stress, immunosuppressant medications, and severe intercurrent illnesses.

The longer one is ill with Lyme, the more likely the illness will be more severe and treatment resistant. The same studies that demonstrated lymphocyte inhibition and lysis from high spirochete loads also demonstrated increased negative effects on the immune system the longer the spirochetes were present. We have seen this clinically, with the ultimate result being full blown Chronic Lyme Disease.

CO-INFECTION

A huge body of research and clinical experience has demonstrated the nearly universal phenomenon in Lyme patients of co-infection with multiple tick-borne pathogens. Significant numbers of Lyme patients have been shown to also carry Babesia species, Ehrlichias, Anaplasmas, Mycoplasmas, Bartonellas and viruses. Rarely, yeast forms have been seen in peripheral blood. Studies have shown that co-infection results in a more severe clinical presentation, with more organ damage, and the pathogens become more difficult to eradicate. It is known that Babesia infection, like Lyme Borreliosis, is immunosuppressive. There are changes in the clinical presentation compared to when each infection is present individually, with different symptoms, and atypical signs. There may be decreased reliability of standard diagnostic tests, and most importantly, there is recognition that chronic, persistent forms of each of these infections do indeed exist. As time goes by, I am convinced that even more pathogens will be found.

Therefore, real, clinical Lyme as we have come to know it, especially the later and more severe presentations, probably represents a mixed infection. I will leave to the reader the implications of how this may explain the discrepancy between laboratory study of pure Borrelia infections, and what front-line physicians have been seeing for years in real patients.

The evaluation of a Lyme patient must begin with testing for all currently known tick borne pathogens. Serological studies for Borrelia, Babesia Bartonella and Ehrlichia should be combined where appropriate with direct antigen assays. Antigen detection tests (antigen capture and PCR) are especially helpful in evaluating the seronegative patient and those still ill or relapsing after therapy. Unfortunately, over a dozen protozoans other than Babesia microti can be found in ticks, yet commercial tests for only B. microti and WA-1 are available at this time, so as in Borrelia, clinical assessment is the primary diagnostic tool. In Ehrlichiosis, test for both the monocytic and granulocytic forms. Many presently uncharacterized Ehrlichia-like organisms can be found in ticks and may not be picked up by currently available assays, so in this illness too, serologies are only an adjunct in making the diagnosis.

Babesia are parasites, and I suggest that if a coinfection is found involving this organism, treat this first, so that subsequent therapy for the other pathogens will be more effective.

COLLATERAL CONDITIONS

Experience has shown that collateral conditions exist in those who have been ill a long time. The evaluation should include testing both for differential diagnosis and for uncovering other subtle abnormalities that may coexist.

Test B12 levels, and be prepared to aggressively treat with parenteral formulations.

Pituitary and other endocrine abnormalities are far more common than generally realized. Evaluate fully, including growth hormone levels. When testing the thyroid, measure free T3 and free T4 levels and TSH. Nuclear scanning and testing for autoantibodies may be necessary.

Activation of the inflammatory cascade has been implicated in blockade of cellular hormone receptors. One example of this is insulin resistance, which may partly account for the dyslipidemia and weight gain that is noted in 80% of chronic Lyme patients. Clinical hypothyroidism can result from receptor blockade and thus hypothyroidism can exist despite normal serum hormone levels. In addition to measuring free T3 and T4 levels, check basal A.M. body temperatures. If hypothyroidism is found, you may need to treat with both T3 and T4 preparations until blood levels of both are normalized.

Tilt table testing is another powerful tool which, just as in CFIDS, may demonstrate neurally mediated hypotension (NMH). NMH can result from autonomic neuropathy and endocrine dyscrasias. If NMH is present, treatment can dramatically lessen fatigue, palpitations and wooziness, and increase stamina. This test should be done by a cardiologist and include Isuprel challenge. This will demonstrate not only if NMH is present, but also the relative contributions of hypovolemia and sympathetic dysfunction. Therapy is based on blood volume expansion (increased sodium and fluid intake and possibly Florinef plus potassium). If not sufficient, beta blockade may be added based on response to the Isuprel challenge.

Magnesium deficiency is very often present and quite severe. Hyperreflexia, muscle twitches, myocardial irritability, poor stamina and recurrent tight muscle spasms are clues to this deficiency. Magnesium is predominantly an intracellular ion, so blood level testing is of little value. Oral preparations are acceptable for maintenance, but most need additional, parenteral dosing: 1 gram IV or IM at least once a week until neuromuscular irritability has cleared.

SPECT scanning of the brain, if done by knowledgeable radiologists using high resolution equipment, will show characteristic abnormalities in Lyme encephalopathy. What these scans demonstrate is cerebral vasculitis, which is the underlying mechanism for much of the symptoms of Lyme. This not only helps with the differential diagnosis, but if done before and after acetazolamide, it will guide in the use of vasodilators, which may clear some cognitive symptoms. Therapy can include acetazolamide, serotonin agonists and even Ginkgo biloba. Therapeutic trials of these may be needed.

Two different researchers have provided evidence that B. burgdorferi, like many other pathogenic bacteria, can produce neurotoxins. Early clinical trials aimed at removing these toxins have proven quite promising. I will discuss this in more detail in a later section.

**LYME BORRELIOSIS
DIAGNOSTIC HINTS**

Lyme is diagnosed clinically, as no currently available test, no matter the source or type, is definitive in ruling in or ruling out infection with these pathogens, or whether these infections are responsible for the patient's symptoms. The entire clinical picture must be taken into account, including a search for concurrent conditions and alternate diagnoses, and other reasons for some of the presenting complaints. Often, much of the diagnostic process in late, disseminated Lyme involves ruling out other illnesses and defining the extent of damage that might require separate evaluation and treatment.

Consideration should be given to tick exposure, rashes (even atypical ones), evolution of typical symptoms in a previously asymptomatic individual, and results of tests for tick-borne pathogens. Another very important factor is response to treatment — presence or absence of Jarisch Herxheimer-like reactions, the classic four-week cycle of waxing and waning of symptoms, and improvement with therapy.

ERYTHEMA MIGRANS

Erythema migrans (EM) is diagnostic of Bb infection, but is present in fewer than half. Even if present, it may go unnoticed by the patient. It is an erythematous, centrifugally expanding lesion that is raised and warm. Sometimes there is mild stinging or pruritus. The EM rash will begin four days to several weeks after the bite, and may be associated with constitutional symptoms. Multiple lesions are present less than 10% of the time, but do represent disseminated disease. Some lesions have an atypical appearance and skin biopsy specimens may be helpful. When an ulcerated or vesicular center is seen, this may represent a mixed infection, involving other organisms besides B. burgdorferi.

After a tick bite, serologic tests (ELISA. IFA, western blots, etc.) are not expected to become positive until several weeks have passed. Therefore, if EM is present, treatment must begin immediately, and one should not wait for results of Borrelia tests. You should not miss the chance to treat early disease, for this is when the success rate is the highest. Indeed, many knowledgeable clinicians will not even order a Borrelia test in this circumstance.

DIAGNOSING LATER DISEASE

When reactive, serologies indicate exposure only and do not directly indicate whether the spirochete is now currently present. Because Bb serologies often give inconsistent results, test at more than one laboratory using, if possible, different methods. The suggestion that two-tiered testing, utilizing an ELISA as a screening tool, followed, if positive, by a confirmatory western blot, is illogical in this illness. The ELISA is not sensitive enough to serve as an adequate screen, and there are many patients with Lyme who test negative by ELISA yet have fully diagnostic western blots. I therefore recommend against using the ELISA. Order IgM and IgG western blots — but be aware that in late disease there may be repeatedly peaking IgM's and therefore a reactive IgM may not differentiate early from late disease, but it does suggest an active infection. When late cases of LB are seronegative, 36% will transiently become seropositive at the completion of successful therapy.

Western blots are reported by showing which bands are reactive. 41KD bands appear the earliest but can cross react with other spirochetes. The 18KD, 23–25KD (Osp C), 31KD (Osp A), 34KD (Osp B), 37KD, 39KD, 83KD and the 93KD bands are the most specific but appear later or may not appear at all. You need to see at least the 41KD and one of the specific bands. 55KD, 60KD, 66KD, and 73KD are nonspecific and nondiagnostic.

PCR tests are now available, and although they are very specific, sensitivity remains poor, possibly less than 30%. This is because Bb causes a deep tissue infection and is only transiently found in body humors. Therefore, just as in routine blood culturing, multiple specimens must be collected to increase yield; a negative result does not rule out infection, but a positive one is significant. You can test whole blood, buffy coat, serum, urine, spinal and other body fluids, and tissue biopsies. Several blood PCRs can be done, or you can run PCRs on whole blood, serum and urine simultaneously at a time of active symptoms. The patient should be antibiotic free for at least six weeks before testing to obtain the highest yield.

Antigen capture is becoming more widely available, and can be done on urine, CSF, and synovial fluid.

Sensitivity is still low, but specificity is high.

Spinal taps are not routinely recommended, as a negative tap does not rule out Lyme. Antibodies to Bb most commonly are found in Lyme meningitis, but are rarely seen in non-meningitic CNS infection, including even advanced encephalopathy. Even in meningitis, antibodies are detected in the CSF in less than 20% of patients with late disease. Therefore, spinal taps are only performed on patients with pronounced neurological manifestations in whom the diagnosis is uncertain, if they are seronegative, or are still significantly symptomatic after completion of treatment. When done, the goal is to rule out other conditions, and to determine if Bb antigens or nucleic acids are present. It is especially important to look for elevated protein and mononuclear cells, which would dictate the need for more aggressive therapy, as well as the opening pressure, which can be elevated and add to headaches, especially in children.

I strongly urge you to biopsy all unexplained skin lesions/rashes and perform PCR and careful histology. You will need to alert the pathologist to look for spirochetes.

DIAGNOSTIC CHECKLIST

To aid the clinician, a workable set of diagnostic criteria was developed with the input of dozens of front line physicians. The resultant document has proven to be extremely useful not only to the clinician, but it also can help clarify the diagnosis for third party payers and utilization review committees.

It is important to note that the CDC's published reporting criteria are for surveillance only, not for diagnosis.

LYME BORRELIOSIS DIAGNOSTIC CRITERIA	RELATIVE VALUE
Tick exposure in an endemic region	1
Historical facts and evolution of symptoms consistent with Lyme	2
Systemic signs & symptoms consistent with Bb infection (other potential diagnoses excluded):	
Single system, e.g., monoarthritis	1
Two or more systems, e.g., monoarthritis and facial palsy	2
Erythema migrans, physician confirmed	7
Acrodermatitis Chronica Atrophicans, biopsy confirmed	7
Seropositivity	3
Seroconversion on paired sera	4
Tissue microscopy, silver stain	3
Tissue microscopy, monoclonal immunofluorescence	4
Culture positivity	4
B. burgdorferi antigen recovery	4
B. burgdorferi DNA/RNA recovery	4

DIAGNOSIS

Lyme Borreliosis Highly Likely	7 or above

I suggest that when using these criteria, you state Lyme Borreliosis is "unlikely," "possible," or "highly likely" based upon the following criteria—then list the criteria.

SYMPTOM CHECKLIST
This is not meant to be used as a diagnostic scheme, but is provided to streamline the office interview. Note the format — complaints referable to specific organ systems are clustered to better display multisystem involvement.

NAME_____

DATE_____

RISK PROFILE (PLEASE CHECK)
Tick infested area ____ Frequent outdoor activities ____
Hiking ____ Fishing ____ Camping ____ Gardening ____
Hunting ____ Ticks noted on pets ____ Other household members with Lyme ____
Do you remember being bitten by a tick? No ____ Yes ____ when _____
Do you remember having the "bull's eye rash?"
No ____ Yes ____
Any other rash? No ____ Yes ____
Have you had any of the following? CIRCLE ALL YES ANSWERS
    Unexplained fevers, sweats, chills, or flushing
    Unexplained weight change (loss or gain — circle one)
    Fatigue, tiredness, poor stamina
    Unexplained hair loss
    Swollen glands: list areas

_____

    Sore throat
    Testicular pain/pelvic pain
    Unexplained menstrual irregularity
    Unexplained milk production; breast pain
    Irritable bladder or bladder dysfunction
    Sexual dysfunction or loss of libido
    Upset stomach or abdominal pain

Change in bowel function (constipation, diarrhea)
Chest pain or rib soreness
Shortness of breath, cough
Heart palpitations, pulse skips, heart block
Any history of a heart murmur or valve prolapse?
Joint pain or swelling: list joints

Stiffness of the joints or back
Muscle pain or cramps
Twitching of the face or other muscles
Headache
Neck creaks and cracks, neck stiffness, neck pain
Tingling, numbness, burning or stabbing sensations, shooting pains, skin hypersensitivity
Facial paralysis (Bell's Palsy)
Eyes/Vision: double, blurry, increased floaters, light sensitivity
Ears/Hearing: buzzing, ringing, ear pain, sound sensitivity
Increased motion sickness, vertigo, poor balance
Lightheadedness, wooziness, unavoidable need to sit or lie down
Tremor
Confusion, difficulty in thinking
Difficulty with concentration, reading
Forgetfulness, poor short term memory, poor attention, problem absorbing new information
Disorientation: getting lost, going to wrong places
Difficulty with speech or writing; word or name block
Mood swings, irritability, depression
Disturbed sleep — too much, too little, fractionated, early awakening
Exaggerated symptoms or worse hangover from alcohol

LYME DISEASE TREATMENT GUIDELINES
LYME BORRELIOSIS
GENERAL INFORMATION

After a tick bite, Bb undergoes rapid hematogenous dissemination, and, for example, can be found within the central nervous system as soon as twelve hours after entering the bloodstream. This is why even early infections require full dose antibiotic therapy with an agent able to penetrate all tissues in concentrations known to be bactericidal to the organism.

It has been shown that the longer a patient had been ill with Bb prior to first definitive therapy, the longer the duration of treatment must be, and the need for more aggressive treatment increases.

More evidence has accumulated indicating the severe detrimental effects of immunosuppressants including steroids in the patient with active B. burgdorferi infection. Never give steroids or any other immunosuppressant to any patient who may even remotely be suffering from Lyme, or serious, permanent damage may result, especially if given for anything greater than a short course. If immunosuppressive therapy is absolutely necessary, then potent antibiotic treatment should begin at least 48 hours prior to the immunosuppressants.

TREATMENT RESISTANCE

Bb contains beta lactamases, which, with some strains, may confer resistance to cephalosporins and penicillins. This is apparently a slowly acting enzyme system, and may be overcome by higher or more continuous drug levels especially when maintained by continuous infusions (cefotaxime) and by depot preparations (benzathine penicillin). Nevertheless, some penicillin and cephalosporin treatment failures do occur and have responded to sulbactam/ampicillin, imipenim, and vancomycin, which act through different cell wall mechanisms than penicillin and the cephalosporins.

There is evidence that B. burgdorferi can remain viable within cells, such as macrophages, lymphocytes, endothelial cells, neurons, and fibroblasts. Bb has been shown to evade the effects of beta lactam antibiotics in vitro by sequestering in these intracellular niches. In addition, Bb can coat itself with host cell membranes, and it secretes a glycoprotein that can encapsulate the organism (an "S-layer"). Because this glycoprotein binds host IgM, it is possible that host protein as well as cell membrane hide Borrelial antigens. In theory at least, these coatings interfere with immune recognition, thus affecting the clearing of Bb, and also cause seronegativity.

There are multiple strains of Borrelia burgdorferi and they vary in their antigen profile and antibiotic susceptibilities. It has also been recognized that B. burgdorferi can exist in at least three different morphologic forms: spirochetal, spheroplast (or l-form), and the recently discovered cystic form.

L-forms and cystic forms do not contain cell walls, and thus beta lactam antibiotics will not affect them. Spheroplasts seem to be susceptible to tetracyclines and some erythromycins, yet the cyst has so far only been proven to be susceptible to metronidazole. Apparently, Bb can shift among the three forms during the course of the infection and cause the varying serologic responses seen over time, including seronegativity. Because of this, it may be necessary to change antibiotic or even prescribe a combination of agents.

Vegetative endocarditis has been associated with Borrelia burgdorferi, but the vegetations may be too small to detect with echocardiography. Keep this in mind when evaluating patients with murmurs, as this may explain why some patients seem to continually relapse after even long courses of antibiotics.

COURSE DURING THERAPY

As the spirochete has a very long generation time (12 to 24 hours in vitro and possibly much longer in living systems) and may have periods of dormancy, during which time antibiotics will not kill the organism, treatment has to be continued for a long period of time to eradicate all the active symptoms and prevent a relapse, especially in late infections. If treatment is discontinued before all symptoms of active infection have cleared, the patient will remain ill and possibly relapse further. In general, early disseminated LB is treated for four to six weeks, and late LB usually requires a minimum of four to six months of continuous treatment. All patients respond differently and therapy must be individualized. It is not uncommon for a patient who has been ill for many years to require open ended treatment regimens; indeed, some patients will require ongoing maintenance therapy to remain well.

Several days after the onset of appropriate antibiotic therapy, symptoms often flare due to lysis of the spirochetes with release of increased amount of antigenic material and possibly bacterial toxins. This is referred to as a Jarish Herxheimer-like reaction. Because it takes 48 to 72 hours of therapy to initiate bacterial killing, the Herxheimer reaction is therefore delayed. This is unlike syphilis, in which these reactions can occur within hours.

It has been observed that symptoms will flare in cycles every four weeks. It is thought that this reflects the organism's cell cycle, with the growth phase occurring once per month (intermittent growth is common in Borrelia species). As antibiotics will only kill bacteria during their growth phase, therapy is designed to bracket at least one whole generation cycle. This is why the minimum treatment duration should be at least four weeks. If the antibiotics are working, over time these flares will lessen in severity and duration. The very occurrence of ongoing monthly cycles indicates that living organisms are still present and that antibiotics should be continued.

With treatment, these monthly symptom flares are exaggerated and presumably represent recurrent Herxheimer-like reactions as Bb enters its vulnerable growth phase then are lysed. For unknown reasons, the worst occurs at the fourth week of treatment. Observation suggest that the more severe this reaction, the higher the germ load, and the more ill the patient. In those with long-standing highly symptomatic disease who are on IV therapy, the week-four flare can be very severe, similar to a serum sickness reaction, and be associated with transient leucopenia and/or elevations in liver enzymes. If this happens, decrease the dose temporarily, or interrupt treatment for several days, then resume with a lower dose. If you are able to continue or resume therapy, then patients continue to improve. Those whose treatment is stopped and not restarted at this point usually will need re-treatment in the future due to ongoing or recurrent symptoms because the infection was not eradicated. Patients on IV therapy who have a strong reaction at the fourth week will need to continue parenteral antibiotics for several months, for when this monthly reaction finally lessens in severity, then oral or IM medications can be substituted. Indeed, it is just this observation that guides the clinician in determining the endpoint of IV treatment. In general, IV therapy is given until there is a clear positive response, then treatment is changed to IM or po until free of signs of active infection for 4 to 8 weeks. Some patients, however, will not respond to IM or po treatment and IV therapy will have to be used throughout. As mentioned earlier, leucopenia may be a sign of persistent Ehrlichiosis, so be sure to look into this.

Repeated treatment failures should alert the clinician to the possibility of an otherwise inapparent immune deficiency, and a workup for this may be advised. Obviously, evaluation for co-infection should be performed, and a search for other or concurrent diagnoses needs to be entertained.

There are three things that will predict treatment failure regardless of which regimen is chosen: Non-compliance, alcohol use on a regular basis, and failure of the patient to obtain proper rest. Advise them to take a break when (or ideally before) the inevitable mid afternoon fatigue sets in.

All patients must keep a carefully detailed daily diary of their symptoms to help us judge the effects of treatment, the presence of the classic four week cycle, and treatment endpoint. One must follow such diaries, temperature readings in late afternoon, physical findings, notes from physical therapists, and cognitive testing to best judge when to change or end antibiotics.

Remember — there currently is no test for cure, so this clinical follow-up assumes a major role in Lyme Disease care.

BORRELIA NEUROTOXIN (With thanks to Dr. Shoemaker)
Two groups have reported evidence that Borrelia, like several

other bacteria, produce neurotoxins. These compounds reportedly can cause many of the symptoms of encephalopathy, cause an ongoing inflammatory reaction manifested as some of the virus-like symptoms common in late Lyme, and also potentially interfere with hormone action by blocking hormone receptors. At this time, there is no assay available to detect whether this compound is present, nor can the amount of toxin be quantified. Indirect measures are currently employed, such as measures of cytokine activation and hormone resistance. A visual contrast sensitivity test (VCS test) reportedly is quite useful in documenting CNS effects of the neurotoxin, and to follow effects of treatment. This test is available at some centers and on the internet.

It has been said that the longer one is ill with Lyme, the more neurotoxin is present in the body. It probably is stored in fatty tissues, and once present, persists for a very long time. This may be because of enterohepatic circulation, where the toxin is excreted via the bile into the intestinal tract, but then is reabsorbed from the intestinal tract back into the blood stream. This forms the basis for treatment.

Synthetic fiber agents, available by prescription for the treatment of high cholesterol, have the ability to bind some bacterial toxins. When take orally in generous amounts, the neurotoxin, present in the intestinal tract, binds to the resin, is trapped, and then excreted. Thus, over several weeks, the level of neurotoxin is depleted and clinical improvement can be seen. Current experience is that improvement is first seen in three weeks, and treatment continues for two to four months. Retreatment is always possible.

Two prescription medications that can bind these toxins include cholestyramine resin (Questran), and Welchol pills. These medications may bind not only toxins but also many drugs and vitamin supplements. Therefore no other oral medications or supplements should be taken from one hour before, to three hours after a dose of one of these fiber agents.

Cholestyramine must be taken four times daily, and Welchol is prescribed at three pills twice daily. While the latter is obviously much simpler to use, it is less effective than cholestyramine. The main side effects are bloating and constipation, best handled with increased fluid intake and gentle laxatives.

LYME DISEASE TREATMENT INFORMATION

There is no universally effective antibiotic for treating LB. The choice of medication used and the dosage prescribed will vary for different people based on multiple factors. These include duration and severity of illness, presence of co-infections, immune deficiencies, prior significant immunosuppressant use while infected, age, weight, gastrointestinal function, blood levels achieved, and patient tolerance. Doses found to be effective clinically are often higher than those recommended in older texts. This is due to deep tissue penetration by Bb, it's presence in the CNS including the eye, within cells, within tendons, and because very few of the many strains of this organism now known to exist have been studied for antibiotic susceptibility. In addition, all animal studies of susceptibility to date have only addressed early disease in models that behave differently than human hosts. Therefore, begin with a regimen appropriate to the setting, and if necessary, modify it over time based upon response.

ANTIBIOTICS

There are several types of antibiotics in general use for Bb treatment. The tetracyclines, including doxycycline and minocycline, are bacteriostatic unless given in high doses. If high blood levels are not attained, treatment failures in early and late disease are common. However, these high doses can be difficult to tolerate. For example, doxycycline can be very effective but only if adequate blood levels are achieved either by high oral doses (300 to 600 mg daily) or by parenteral administration.

Penicillins are bactericidal. As would be expected in managing an infection with a gram negative organism such as Bb, amoxicillin has been shown to be more effective than oral penicillin V. Because of its short half-life and need for high levels, amoxicillin is usually administered along with probenecid. Since blood levels are extremely variable they should be measured.

Cephalosporins must be of advanced generation: first generation drugs are rarely effective, and second generation drugs are comparable to amoxicillin and doxycycline both in-vitro and in-vivo. Third generation agents are currently the most effective of the cephalosporins because of their very low MBC's (0.06 for ceftriaxone) and they have been shown to be effective in penicillin and tetracycline failures. Cefuroxime axetil (Ceftin), a second generation agent, is also effective against staph and thus is useful in treating atypical erythema migrans that may represent a mixed infection, containing some of the more common skin pathogens in addition to Bb.

When choosing a third generation cephalosporin, there are several points to remember: Ceftriaxone has 95% biliary excretion and can crystallize in the biliary tree with resultant colic and possible cholecystitis. GI excretion results in a large impact on gut flora. Biliary and superinfection problems with ceftriaxone can be lessened if this drug is given in interrupted courses, such as three to five days in a row each week. More recently, chenodeoxycholic acid, used to dissolve gallstones, is being prescribed along with ceftriaxone as prophylaxis. Cefotaxime is less convenient to administer because of the need for either multiple daily doses or continuous infusions, but as it has only 5% biliary excretion, it never causes biliary concretions, and may have less impact on gut flora. It is the experience of some clinicians that cefotaxime can be even more efficacious if given as a continuous infusion, rather than in interrupted doses.

Erythromycin has been shown to be almost ineffective as monotherapy. The advanced macrolides and azalides such as azithromycin and clarithromycin can be difficult to tolerate orally due to their tendency to promote yeast overgrowth and poor GI tolerance at the high doses needed. As they have impressively low MBCs and do concentrate in tissues and penetrate cells, they theoretically should be ideal agents. However, initial clinical results were disappointing, especially with oral azithromycin. It has been suggested that when Bb is within a cell, it is held within a vacuole and bathed in fluid of low pH, and this acidity may inactivate this class of antibiotics. Therefore, they are administered concurrently with hydroxychloroquine or amantadine, which raise vacuolar pH, rendering these antibiotics more effective. It is not known whether this same technique will make erythromycin a more effective antibiotic in LB. Another alternative is to administer azithromycin parenterally. Results are excellent, but expect to see abrupt Jarisch-Herxheimer reactions.

Metronidazole (Flagyl) is commonly used in select patients with treatment resistant, chronic Lyme. When present in a hostile environment, such as growth medium lacking some nutrients, or spinal fluid, or serum with certain antibiotics added, Bb will change into a cystic form. This cyst seems to be able to remain dormant, but when placed into an environment more favorable to its growth, the cyst can open, and an intact spirochete emerges. The conventional antibiotics used for Lyme, such as the penicillins, cephalosporins, etc. do not kill the cystic form of Bb. Furthermore, the cyst lacks the usual surface antigens found on the spirochete (these are the markers detected by ELISAs and western blots). This may be another reason for the chronically sick Lyme patient remaining seronegative.

There is evidence that metronidazole will kill the cystic form. This fits with the now well known clinical observations that metronidazole can be remarkably effective for many chronic Lyme patients. However, this medication apparently has no effect on intact spirochetes. Therefore, the trend now is to treat the chronically infected patient who has resistant disease by combining metronidazole with one or two other antibiotics to target all forms of Bb. Because there is laboratory evidence that tetracyclines may inhibit the effect of metronidazole, this class of medication may not be as useful as others in these two- and three-drug regimens. There have been some recent reports that Bb does not contain genes that would confer susceptibility to metronidazole. However, this clearly does not fit with in vitro and a large body of clinical data, which have demonstrated the usefulness of this agent in the Lyme patient. Perhaps we do not have all the genetic information needed to dismiss the use of this agent. Once again, real world experience is one step ahead of bench research.

Important precautions:

Pregnancy while on metronidazole is not advised, as there is a risk of birth defects.

No alcohol consumption! A severe, "antabuse" reaction will occur, consisting of severe nausea, flushing, headache, and other unpleasant symptoms.

Metronidazole is potentially neurotoxic. Peripheral neuropathy may result. Therefore, breaks in treatment are commonly prescribed, such as using this agent every other week.

Yeast overgrowth is especially common. A strict anti-yeast regimen must be followed.

VERY severe Herxheimer-like reactions are seen in the more ill patient during the first week of therapy, and again four weeks later.

COMBINATION THERAPY

This consists of using two or more dissimilar antibiotics simultaneously. There are several reasons for this. Combinations should utilize dissimilar antibiotics for antibiotic synergism, to better compensate for differing killing profiles and sites of action of the individual medications, and to cover the three known morphologic forms of Bb. The idea is to work in body fluids and in deep tissues, outside and within cells, and effect killing by different mechanisms for synergism. An example is a combination of amoxicillin and clarithromycin. Note how complimentary these two are for treating infection with Bb. GI intolerance and yeast superinfections are the biggest drawbacks to this type of treatment. However, these complications can often be prevented or easily treated, and the clinically observed benefits of this type of regimen clearly have outweighed these problems in selected patients.

PULSE THERAPY

This consists of administering antibiotics (usually parenteral ones) two to three days in a row per week. The efficacy of this regimen is based on the fact that it takes 48 to 72 hours of continuous bactericidal antibiotic levels to kill the spirochete, yet it will take longer than the four to five days between pulses for the spirochetes to recover. This allows for several advantages:

- Dosages are doubled (ie: cefotaxime, 12 g daily), increasing efficacy
- More toxic medications can be used with increased safety (ie: vancomycin)
- May be effective when conventional, daily regimens have failed.
- IV access may be easier or more tolerable
- More agreeable lifestyle for the patient
- Often less costly than daily regimens

Note that this type of treatment is expected to continue for a minimum of ten weeks, and often must continue beyond twenty weeks. As with all Lyme treatments, specific dosing and scheduling must be tailored to the individual patient's clinical picture based upon the treating physician's best clinical judgment.

MONITORING THERAPY

Drug levels are measured, where possible, to confirm adequate dosing. The regimen may have to be modified to optimize the dose, and again at any time major changes in the treatment regimen occur. With parenteral therapy, CBC and chem/liver panels are done at least twice each month, especially during symptom flares, with urinalysis and protime monitored monthly.

INDICATORS FOR PARENTERAL THERAPY

The following are guidelines only and are not meant to be absolute. It is based on retrospective study of over 600 patients with late Lyme disease.

- Illness for greater than one year
- Prior immunosuppressive therapy
- Major neurological involvement
- Active synovitis with high sedimentation rate
- Elevated protein or cells in the CSF

ANTIBIOTIC CHOICES
ORAL THERAPY
Always check blood levels when using agents marked with an *, and adjust dose to achieve a peak level in the mid- teens and a trough greater than five. Because of this, the doses listed below may have to be raised. Consider Doxycycline first due to concern for Ehrlichia.

*Amoxicillin	Adults: 1g q8h plus probenecid 500mg q8h; doses up to 6 grams daily are often needed
	Pregnancy: 1g q6h and adjust
	Children: 50 mg/kg/day divided into q8h doses
*Doxycycline	Adults: 100 mg qid with food; doses of up to 600 mg daily are often needed, as doxycycline is only effective at high blood levels.
	Not for children or in pregnancy.
	If levels are too low at tolerated doses, give parenterally.
*Cefuroxime axetil	Oral alternative that may be effective in amoxicillin and doxycycline failures. Useful in EM rashes co-infected with common skin pathogens.
	Adults and pregnancy: 1g q12h and adjust.
	Children: 125 to 500 mg q12h based on weight.
Tetracycline	Adults only, and not in pregnancy. 500 mg tid to qid
Erythromycin	Poor response and not recommended.

Clarithromycin	Adults: 500 to 1000 mg q12h. Add hydroxychloroquine, 200–400 mg/d or amantadine 100–200 mg/d.
	Cannot be used in pregnancy or in younger children
Azithromycin	Adults: 500 to 1200 mg/d.
	Adolescents: 250 to 500 mg/d.
	Add hydroxychloroquine, 200–400 mg/d, or amantadine 100–200 mg/d
	Cannot be used in pregnancy.
	Oral azithromycin is not as effective as clarithromycin.
Augmentin	Cannot exceed three tablets daily due to the clavulanate, thus is given with amoxicillin.
	This combination can be effective when Bb beta lactamase is felt to be present.
Chloramphenicol	Not recommended as not proven and potentially toxic.
Metronidazole (see text)	500 to 1500 mg daily in divided doses. Adults only.

PARENTERAL THERAPY

Ceftriaxone	Risk of biliary sludging can be minimized with intermittent breaks in therapy (ie: infuse five or less days in a row per week).
	Adults and pregnancy: 2g q12h, four days in a row each week.
	Children: 75 mg/kg/day up to 2g/day
Cefotaxime	Comparable efficacy to ceftriaxone; no biliary complications.
	Adults and pregnancy: 2g q8h; may dose as high as 12g daily. Suggest a continuous infusion.
	Children: 90 to 180 mg/kg/day dosed q6h (preferred) or q8h, not to exceed 12 g daily.
*Doxycycline	Requires central line as is caustic. Surprisingly effective, probably because higher overall, and spiked blood levels when given parenterally.
	Always measure blood levels.
	Adults: 400 mg q24h and adjust based on levels.
	Cannot be used in pregnancy or in younger children.
Azithromycin	Requires central line as is caustic.
	Dose: 500 to 1000 mg daily in adolescents and adults.
Penicillin G	IV penicillin G is minimally effective and not recommended.

Benzathine penicillin	Surprisingly effective IM alternative to oral therapy.
	May need to begin at lower doses as strong, prolonged (6 or more week) Herxheimer-like reactions have been observed.
	Adults: 1.2 million U three times per week (higher doses with large body habitus)
	Adolescents: 300,000 to 2.4 million U weekly.
	May be used in pregnancy.

Poorly studied but anecdotally effective

Vancomycin	Observed to be one of the best drugs in treating Lyme, but potential toxicity limits its use. It is a perfect candidate for pulse therapy to minimize these concerns.
	Use standard doses and confirm levels.

Imipenim and Unisyn	Similar in efficacy to cefotaxime, but often works when cephalosporins have failed. Must be given q6 to q8 hours.
Cefuroxime	Useful but not demonstrably better than ceftriaxone or cefotaxime.
Ampicillin IV	More effective than penicillin G. Must be given q6 hours.

TREATMENT CATEGORIES

PROPHYLAXIS of high risk groups — education and preventive measures. Antibiotics are not given.

TICK BITES — Embedded Deer Tick With No Signs or Symptoms of Lyme (see appendix)

Decide to treat based on the type of tick, whether it came from an endemic area and percent infected, how it was removed, and length of attachment (nymphs: at least one day; adults: anecdotally, as little as four hours). The risk of transmission is greater if the tick is engorged, or of it was removed improperly allowing the tick's contents to spill into the bite wound. High risk bites are treated as follows (remember the possibility of coinfection!):

Adults: Oral therapy for 21 days.

Pregnancy: Amoxicillin 1000 mg q6h for 6 weeks. Test for Babesia, Bartonella and Ehrlichia.
Alternative: Cefuroxime axetil 1000 mg q12h for 6 weeks.

Young Children: Oral therapy for 21 days.

EARLY LOCALIZED — Single erythema migrans with no constitutional symptoms:

Adults: oral therapy for 6 weeks.

Pregnancy: 1st and 2nd trimesters: IV X 21 days then oral X 6 weeks

3rd trimester: Oral therapy X 6 weeks.

Any trimester — test for Babesia, Bartonella, and Ehrlichia

Children: oral therapy for 6 weeks.

DISSEMINATED DISEASE — Multiple lesions, constitutional symptoms, lymphadenopathy, or any other manifestations of dissemination.

EARLY DISSEMINATED — Milder symptoms present for less than one year and not complicated by immune deficiency or prior immunosuppressive treatment:

Adults: Oral therapy until no active disease for 4 weeks (4–6 months typical)

Pregnancy: As in localized disease, but duration as above. Treat throughout pregnancy, and do not breast feed.

Children: Oral therapy with duration based upon clinical response.

PARENTERAL ALTERNATIVES for more ill patients and those unresponsive to or intolerant of oral medications:

Adults and children: IV therapy for at least 6 weeks (until clearly improved).

Follow with oral therapy or IM benzathine penicillin until no active disease for 6–8 weeks.

IV may have to be resumed if oral or IM therapy fails.

Pregnancy: IV then oral therapy as above.

LATE DISSEMINATED — Present greater than one year, more severely ill patients, and those with prior significant steroid therapy or any other cause of impaired immunity:

Adults and pregnancy: Extended IV therapy (10 or more weeks), then oral or IM, if effective, to same endpoint.

Children: IV therapy for 6 or more weeks, then oral or IM follow up as above.

CHRONIC LYME DISEASE

By definition, this category consists of patients with active infection, of a more prolonged duration, and most likely have higher spirochete loads, weaker defense mechanisms, possibly more virulent or resistant strains, and probably are significantly co-infected. Neurotoxins may also be significant in these patients. Search for and treat concurrent illnesses including viruses, chlamydias, and mycoplasmas. These patients require a full evaluation for all of these problems, and each abnormality must be addressed.

This group will most likely need parenteral therapy, especially high dose, pulsed therapy, and antibiotic combinations, including metronidazole. Antibiotic therapy will need to continue for many months, and the antibiotics may have to be changed periodically to break plateaus in recovery. Be vigilant for treatment-related problems such as antibiotic-associated colitis, yeast overgrowth, intravenous catheter complications, and abnormalities in blood counts and chemistries.

If treatment can be continued long term, then a remarkable degree of recovery is possible. However, attention must be paid to all treatment modalities for such a recovery — not only antibiotics, but rehab programs, nutritional supplements, enforced rest, low carbohydrate, high fiber diets, attention to food sensitivities, avoidance of stress, abstinence from caffeine and alcohol, and absolutely no immunosuppressants, even local doses of steroids (intra articular injections, for example).

Unfortunately, not all patients with chronic Lyme disease will fully recover and treatment may not eradicate the active Borrelia infection. Such individuals may have to be maintained on open-ended, ongoing antibiotic therapy, for they repeatedly relapse after antibiotics are stopped. Maintenance antibiotic therapy is thus mandatory.

SAFETY

Nearly two decades of experience in treating thousands of patients with Lyme has proven that therapy as described above, although intense, is generally well tolerated. The most common adverse reaction seen is allergy to probenecid. In addition, yeast superinfections are seen, but these are generally easily recognized and managed. The induction of Clostridium difficile toxin production is seen most commonly with ceftriaxone, but can occur with any of the antibiotic regimens mentioned in this document. However, pulsed dose therapy and regular use of the lactobacillus preparations seems to be helpful in controlling yeast and antibiotic related colitis, as the number of cases of C. difficile in Lyme patients is low when these guidelines are followed.

When using central intravenous lines including PICC lines (peripherally inserted central catheters), if ANY line problems arise, it is recommended that the line be pulled for patient safety. Salvage attempts (urokinase, repairing holes) are often ineffective and may not be safe.

Please advise all patients who take the tetracyclines of skin and eye sensitivity to sunlight and the proper precautions, and advise birth control if appropriate. When doxycycline is given parenterally, do not refreeze the solution prior to use!

Remember, years of experience with chronic antibiotic therapy in other conditions, including rheumatic fever, acne, gingivitis, recurrent otitis, recurrent cystitis, COPD, bronchiectasis, and others have not revealed any consistent dire consequences as a result of such medication use. Indeed, the very real consequences of untreated, chronic persistent infection by B. burgdorferi can be far worse than the potential consequences of this treatment.

CO-INFECTIONS IN LYME
PIROPLASMOSIS (Babesiosis)
GENERAL INFORMATION

Piroplasms are not bacteria, they are protozoans. Therefore, they will not be eradicated by any of the currently used Lyme treatment regimens. Therein lies the significance of co-infections — if a Lyme patient has been extensively treated yet is still ill, suspect a co-infection.

Babesia infection is becoming more commonly recognized, especially in patients who already have Lyme Disease. It has been published that as many as 66% of Lyme patients show evidence of co-infection with Babesia. It has also been reported that Babesial infections can range in severity from mild, subclinical infection, to fulminant, potentially life-threatening illness. The more severe presentations are more likely to be seen in immunocompromised and elderly patients. Milder infections are often missed because the symptoms are incorrectly ascribed to Lyme. Babesial infections, even mild ones, may recrudesce and cause severe illness. This phenomenon has been reported to occur at any time, even up to several years after the initial infection. Furthermore, asymptomatic carriers pose risks: to the blood supply as this infection has been reported to be passed on by blood transfusion, and to the unborn child from an infected mother as it can be transmitted *in utero*. Some quotes from the literature:

Krause, PJ. Spielman, A, Telford, SR et.al. *Persistent parasitemia after acute Babesiosis* N Engl J Med 1998. 339:160

"The clinical spectrum of human Babesiosis ranges from an apparently silent infection to a fulminant malaria-like disease."

"When left untreated, silent Babesial infection may persist for months to years."

"Silent infections, which occur in about a third of infected people, may recrudesce."

"Babesial infection may recrudesce after many months of asymptomatic parasitemia."

"Although parasites were initially detected microscopically in the blood of two of the untreated subjects, and all of the treated subjects, none could be found a week after the onset of illness."

"Persistent symptoms of Babesiosis accompanied persistent blood-borne Babesial DNA."

"The persistence of seroreactivity increasingly correlated with the persistence of Babesial DNA."

"In those with only subtle symptoms, Babesiosis often remains undiagnosed."

"Furthermore, physicians tend not to recognize Babesial infection in those who are co-infected with the agent of Lyme Disease, because Babesial symptoms tend to be ascribed to Lyme Disease."

"Physicians caring for patients with moderate to severe Lyme disease should consider obtaining diagnostic tests for Babesiosis and possibly other tick-borne pathogens... especially in patients experiencing "atypical Lyme disease" or patients in whom the response to antibiotic treatment is delayed or absent."

Krause, PJ, Telford, SR, Spielman, A, et.al. *Concurrent Lyme disease and Babesiosis*. JAMA 1996. 275 (21):1657

"Subjects with evidence of both infections reported a greater array of symptoms than those infected by the spirochete or piroplasm alone."

"Co-infection generally results in more intense acute illness and a more prolonged convalescence than accompany either infection alone."

"Spirochete DNA was evident more often and remained in the circulation longer in co-infected subjects than in those experiencing either infection alone."

"Co-infection might also synergize spirochete-induced lesions in human joints, heart and nerves."

"Babesial infections may impair human host defense mechanisms"

"The possibility of concomitant Babesial infection should be considered when moderate to severe Lyme Disease has been diagnosed."

SYMPTOMS

In milder forms, symptoms may include a vague sense of imbalance without true vertigo, headache, mild encephalopathy, fatigue, sweats, air hunger and occasionally cough. When present as a co-infection with Lyme, initial symptoms of the illness are often more acute and severe. Suggestions of co-infection include the above symptoms, but the headaches are more severe, and encephalopathy is out of proportion to the other Borrelia symptoms. The fulminant presentations include high fevers, shaking chills and hemolysis, and can be fatal.

DIAGNOSTIC TESTS

Diagnostic tests are insensitive and problematic. There are at least thirteen Babesial forms found in ticks, yet we can currently only test for B. microti and WA-1 with our serologic and nuclear tests. Standard blood smears reportedly are reliable for only the first two weeks of infection, thus are not useful for diagnosing later infections and milder ones including carrier states where the germ load is too low to be detected.

Krause, PJ, Telford, SR, Spielman, A, et.al. *Concurrent Lyme disease and Babesiosis*. JAMA 1996. 275 (21):1660

> "As is common in the case of Babesial infections, parasites frequently cannot be seen in blood films."

Therefore, multiple diagnostic test methods are available and each have their own benefits and limitations and often several tests must be done. Be prepared to treat based on clinical presentation, even with negative tests.

SEROLOGY

Unlike Lyme, Babesia titers can reflect infection status. Thus, persistently positive titers or western blots suggest persistent infection.

PCR

This is more sensitive than smears for B. microti, but will not detect other species.

ENHANCED SMEAR

This utilizes buffy coat, prolonged scanning (up to three hours per sample!) and digital photography through custom-made microscopes. Although more sensitive than standard smears, infections can still be missed. The big advantage is that it will display multiple species, not just B. microti.

FLUORESCENT IN-SITU HYBRIDIZATION ASSAY (FISH)

This technique is also a form of blood smear. It is said to be 100-fold more sensitive than standard smears for B. microti, because instead of utilizing standard, ink-based stains, it uses a fluorescent-linked RNA probe and ultraviolet light. The Babesial organisms are then much easier to spot when the slides are scanned. The disadvantage is that currently only B. microti is detected.

TREATMENT

Treating Babesia infections had always been difficult, because the therapy that had been recommended until 1998 consisted of a combination of clindamycin plus quinine. Published reports and clinical experience have shown this regimen to be unacceptable, as nearly half of patients so treated have had to abandon treatment due to serious side effects, many of which were disabling. Furthermore, even in patients who could tolerate these drugs, there was a failure rate approaching 50%.

Krause, PJ. Spielman, A, Telford, SR et.al.. *Persistent parasitemia after acute Babesiosis* N Engl J Med 1998. 339:162

> "Of the treated subjects, almost half had symptoms that were consistent with reactions to quinine, including hearing loss, tinnitus, hypotension, and such gastrointestinal symptoms as anorexia, vomiting, and diarrhea."

> "Although treatment with clindamycin and quinine reduces the duration of parasitemia, infection may persist and recrudesce and side effects are common."

Because of these dismal statistics, the current regimen of choice for Babesiosis is the combination of atovaquone plus azithromycin. This combination was initially studied in animals, and then applied to Humans with good success, because when atovaquone was used alone, resistance developed in 20% of cases, but reportedly did not occur when azithromycin was added. Fewer than 5% of patients have to halt treatment due to side effects, and the success rate is clearly better than that of clindamycin plus quinine.

The duration of treatment with atovaquone plus azithromycin for Babesiosis varies depending on the degree of infection, duration of illness before diagnosis, the health and immune status of the patient, and whether the patient is co-infected with Borrelia burgdorferi. Typically, a three-week course is prescribed for acute cases, while chronic, longstanding infections with significant morbidity and co-infection will require several months of therapy. Relapses have occurred, and retreatment is occasionally needed.

Problems during therapy include diarrhea, mild nausea, the

expense of atovaquone (over $600.00 per bottle — enough for three weeks of treatment), and rarely, a temporary yellowish discoloration of the vision. Regular blood counts, liver panels and amylase levels are recommended during any prolonged course of therapy. Patients who are not cured with this regimen can be retreated but with higher doses, as this has proven effective in many of my patients. Artemesia (a non-prescription herb) may be added, but is not effective when used alone. Metronidazole can also be added to increase efficacy, but there is minimal clinical data on how much more effective this regimen is.

EHRLICHIOSIS
GENERAL INFORMATION

While it is true that this illness can have a fulminant presentation, and may even become fatal if not treated, milder forms do exist, as does chronic low-grade infection, especially when other tick-borne organisms are present. The potential transmission of Ehrlichia during tick bites is the main reason why doxycycline is now the first choice in treating tick bites and early Lyme, before serologies can become positive. When present alone or co-infecting with B. burgdorferi, persistent leukopenia is an important clue. Thrombocytopenia and elevated liver enzymes are less common, but likewise should not be ignored. Headaches, myalgias, and ongoing fatigue seem to relate to this illness, but are extremely difficult to separate from symptoms caused by Bb.

DIAGNOSTIC TESTING

Testing is problematic with Ehrlichia, similar to the situation with Babesiosis. More species are known to be present in ticks than can be tested for with clinically available serologies and PCRs. In addition, serologies and PCRs are of unknown sensitivity and specificity. Standard blood smears for direct visualization of organisms in leukocytes are of low yield. Enhanced smears using buffy coats significantly raises sensitivity and will indicate a wider variety of species. Despite this, infection can be missed, so clinical diagnosis remains the primary diagnostic tool. Again, consider this diagnosis in a Lyme Borreliosis (LB) patient not responding well to therapy.

TREATMENT
Standard treatment consists of Doxycycline, 200 mg daily for two to four weeks. Higher doses, parenteral therapy, and longer treatment durations may be needed based on the duration and severity of illness, and whether immune defects or extreme age is present. However, there are reports of treatment failure even when higher doses and long duration treatment with doxycycline is given. In such cases, consideration may be given for adding rifampin, 600 mg daily, to the regimen.

BARTONELLA
Bartonella henselae, the agent of cat scratch disease, has been found in Ixodid ticks and as a co-infection in patients with Lyme Disease. With co-infection, symptoms of Bartonella are almost impossible to distinguish from Lyme, but may include lymphadenopathy, splenomegaly, hepatomegaly, headache, encephalopathy, somnolence, flu-like malaise, weight loss, sore throat, and a papular or angiomatous rash. In acute cases, there can be hemolysis with anemia, high fever, weakened immune response, jaundice, abnormal liver enzymes, and myalgias. Endocarditis and myocarditis have been reported. More severe infections are associated with immune deficiency and possibly occurrence of opportunistic infections. As in Lyme Disease and Babesiosis, Bartonella may be transmitted to the fetus in the infected pregnant patient.
Diagnostic tests include serology, blood and CSF PCR, and biopsy of skin lesions and lymph nodes.
In the co-infected Lyme patient, eradication may be difficult. Many antibiotic agents have been reported to be effective, including cephalosporins, fluoroquinolones, erythromycins, gentamicin, rifampin and streptomycin. In practice, these patients seem to do best with a combination regimen that utilizes agents that can penetrate cells. Typical combinations include an erythromycin, plus a fluoroquinolone or rifampin.

Treatment progress is most commonly assessed by PCR post treatment and serial titers.

NUTRITIONAL SUPPLEMENTS IN DISSEMINATED LYME DISEASE

Studies on patients with chronic illnesses such as Lyme and Chronic Fatigue have demonstrated that some of the late symptoms are related to cellular damage and deficiencies in certain essential nutrients. Double blinded, placebo controlled studies, and in one case direct assay of biopsy specimens have proven the value of some of the supplements listed. Some are required, while others are optional — see below. They are listed in order of importance.

The quality of supplements used is often more important than the dose. In fact, "mega doses" are not recommended. Instead, seek out, if possible, pharmaceutical grade products, especially if USP certified. Pharmanex brand products are recommended because they fit these criteria. In the list below, it is indicated whether the product should be gotten from Pharmanex, or whether a different source or generic substitute is OK. To order Pharmanex brand products, call 1-800-487-1000 and give the following US reference # 9256681.

BASIC DAILY REGIMEN

ACIDOPHILUS (required when on antibiotics)
Essential daily supplement to maintain the normal balance of bowel flora, especially if on antibiotics, or if gastrointestinal disturbances are present. Always try to get enteric coated, milk-free acidophilus. The best kinds are frozen or refrigerated to ensure potency. Take two with each meal.

MULTI-VITAMIN (required)
I recommend the Life Pack family of multivitamins. These are unique supplements — Pharmaceutical grade and USP certified, they are the only products clinically proven in double-blinded, placebo controlled crossover studies to quench free radicals and raise antioxidant levels in the blood and lipids. Choose LifePak for males under 40, LifePak Women for hormonally active women, and LifePak Prime for

postmenopausal women and for men over 40. They are available through Pharmanex. Continue long term.

CO-Q10 (ubiquinone) — **required if not taking the prescription drug atovaquone (Mepron)**

Deficiencies have been related to poor function of the heart, limitations of stamina, gum disease, and poor resistance to infections. Heart biopsy studies in Lyme patients indicated that they should take between 200 and 300mg daily of standard CoQ 10, or 90 mg of the well absorbed, highly purified, crystalline CoQ 10 product sold by Pharmanex, (surprisingly, the Pharmanex brand is far less expensive than the generic). The body will manufacture its own CoQ 10 when the original illness is controlled, but only if stimulated by aggressive exercise. Therefore, use this supplement until the patient is feeling well and exercising regularly.

VITAMIN B (required)

Clinical studies demonstrated the need for supplement vitamin B in infections with Borrelia, to help clear neurological symptoms. Take one 50 mg B-complex capsule daily. If neuropathy is severe, an additional 50 to 100 mg of B6 daily may be helpful. Generics are OK.

MAGNESIUM (required)

Magnesium supplementation is very helpful for the tremors, twitches, cramps, muscle soreness, heart skips and weakness. It may also help in energy level and cognition. The best source is magnesium L-lactate dehydrate ("Mag-tab SR," sold by Niche Pharmaceuticals [1-800-677-0355], and available at Wal-Mart). DO NOT rely on "cal-mag," calcium plus magnesium combination tablets, as they are not well absorbed. Take at least one to two tablet twice daily. Higher doses may cause diarrhea, and you should check with your physician before using more than this. In some cases, injections or intravenous doses may be necessary. Continue long term.

ESSENTIAL FATTY ACIDS (required)

Studies show that when EFAs are taken regularly, statistically significant improvements in fatigue, aches weakness, vertigo, dizziness, memory, concentration and depression are likely. There are two broad classes: GLA (omega-6 oils) and

EPA (omega-3 oils), derived respectively from plant and fish oils. This is what to take:

Plant Oils: borage oil, evening primrose oil, or black currant seed oil (choose one). Do NOT use Flax seed oil!

Fish Oil: Omega-3 (Fish Oil) capsules, 1000 mg per capsule. Use "Optimum Omega" by Pharmanex, if a higher quality product is desired, or to minimize the "fishy" aftertaste.

RECOMMENDATION: four plant oil capsules and four fish oil capsules daily, taken with meals. Continue for three to four months then try to taper down the dose.

OPTIONAL SUPPLEMENTS FOR SPECIAL CIRCUMSTANCES

CORDYMAX (optional)

Cordyceps is a well-known herb from Tibet and has been shown in clinical studies to improve stamina, fatigue, and enhance lung and antioxidant function. It increases mitochondrial ATP levels and also raises superoxide dismutase levels. The positive effects can be so dramatic, I strongly urge all people with fatigue to try this. Available only from Pharmanex as "CordyMax."

METHYLCOBALAMIN (Methyl B12) (optional)

This is a prescription drug available only from compounding pharmacies. It is related to vitamin B12 and has several documented benefits: it helps to heal damage to the nervous system, enhances diminished T-cell function, can restore the normal diurnal cycle, and can help with memory and cognition. Methyl B12 must injected into the muscle as it will not be absorbed if swallowed or used sublingually. Dose ranges from 25 to 50 mg daily, based on weight.

REISHI MAX (optional)

This enhanced extract from cracked spores of the reishi mushroom has been shown in clinical studies to augment function of the Natural Killer Cells and macrophages. Take two a day for maintenance, and four a day in disease states. Available only from Pharmanex.

ECHINACEA (optional)

May be helpful in fighting acute and chronic viral illnesses. Choose a pharmaceutical grade brand ("Immune Formula" by Pharmanex), and do not use the liquid form as this contains alcohol. Do not take daily on a long-term basis, as the benefit may wear off. For a chronic illness, double the usual daily dose but take in cycles — use daily three weeks on, one week off each month.

BIO-GINKGO (optional)

The most effective ginkgo brand in my experience — pharmaceutical grade, and very high potency to assure full bioavailability. Available only from Pharmanex. Ginkgo has been shown to increase blood flow to many organs, including the brain. Patients report clearer thinking and better memory. Be aware that this brand is strong — start with a low dose, then increase every few days or a pressure-type, vascular headache may result from all the increased circulation.

GLUCOSAMINE (optional)

Can be of long term benefit to the joints. Do not be misled into buying a product that also contains chondroitin, as this chemical does not add anything, but it can make the product more expensive. Look for a product that contains the herb Boswellia serrata — this is a non-irritative anti-inflammatory. Although many generics exist, the Pharmanex product, "Cartilage Formula," has the right ingredients and is of proven efficacy. Expect improvement only over time (several weeks), but plan to use this indefinitely to maintain joint health.

CREATINE (optional)

Creatine has been shown to be of benefit in neuromuscular degenerative diseases such as Lou Gherig's Disease (ALS) and can be very helpful in supporting low blood pressure, as in NMH. Important: To use this safely, you must have an adequate fluid intake. The creatine product should contain taurine, an amino acid needed to enhance creatine absorption, plus some carbohydrate to aid creatine entry into muscle. You will need a 20 gram loading dose for the first five days, then 4 to 10 grams daily maintenance. Try "Cell Tech" from the Vitamin Shop, and follow label directions.

MILK THISTLE (optional)

Useful to support liver function. Take 175 mg three times daily — use an 80% Silymarin extract.

MUSCLE FIX (optional)
This blend of nutrients from Pharmanex really helps sore, tight muscles. Must be taken on an empty stomach — either two, twice daily between meals, or four at bedtime. Can be used intermittently as needed, or daily.

LYME DISEASE REHABILITATION
Those with long-standing tick borne illnesses end up in poor physical condition. **Even with successful treatment of the infections, chronic Lyme patients will not return to normal unless they pursue a formal program of therapeutic exercise, as outlined below**.
In late stage disease, many negative effects to the body are occurring: muscles atrophy, and to some degree, the heart muscle also suffers, as do the joints, tendons, nerves, etc. The percent fat content of the body as a whole rises, the cholesterol rises, and the balance between HDL and LDL becomes less favorable. In at least 80% of the patients, significant weight gain occurs.
Because of the extreme fatigue and body pain, many Lyme sufferers end up spending inordinate amounts of time in bed, and get far less exercise than they did before they became ill. This begins a debilitating downward spiral that can be very difficult to reverse.
As a result, Lyme patients are stiff, weak, tired, have poor stamina, and are at increased risk for cardiovascular disease and diabetes. Antibiotic treatment alone cannot correct these effects. Therefore, it is necessary to prescribe physical therapy, the extent of which depends on an individual patients' condition, followed by a graded exercise program.
The earliest phase involves multiple modalities (massage, heat, TENS, MENS, ultrasound, etc.) and aggressive range of motion exercises supervised by a physical therapist, to relieve discomfort and to promote better sleep and flexibility. The goal of physical therapy is to prepare the patient for the required, gym-based exercise program. This starts with stretching and mild muscular toning. Then, the program must expand to include muscular conditioning and strengthening, ideally under the supervision of a credentialed exer-

cise physiologist. "Body sculpture" classes are ideal. Aerobics are **not** recommended until the patient has fully recovered.

This is the time for the very best of health habits. I recommend light, low fat food, high in fiber, with high quality nutritional value, minimal amounts of starch and other simple carbohydrates, absolute abstention from alcohol, elimination of caffeine, and if applicable, a serious commitment to weight loss. Consider testing for food hypersensitivities and recommending books that outline "arthritis diets," as they can help some patients.

Cessation of smoking is extremely important and must be addressed immediately.

As written orders for physical therapy are required to initiate the program, an example of the format of a typical prescription for Lyme rehabilitation follows.

LYME REHAB — PHYSICAL THERAPY PRESCRIPTION

NAME _____

D.O.B._____

DATE _____

Please enroll this patient in a program of therapy to rehabilitate him/her from the effects of Lyme Disease. If necessary, begin with classic physical therapy, then progress when appropriate to a **whole body** conditioning program. Such therapy must **be graded, carefully individualized, and be performed on a one-on-one basis**, at least initially, to ensure the maximal amount of supervision and guidance.

THERAPEUTIC GOALS (to be achieved in order as the patient's ability allows):

PHYSICAL THERAPY (if needed):

Relieve pain and muscle spasms utilizing multiple modalities as available and as indicated: massage, heat, ultrasound, TENS, "micro amp", etc.

Increase mobility while protecting damaged and weakened joints, tendons, and ligaments, to increase range of motion and relieve stiffness.

Physical therapy alone is not enough. The role of physical therapy here is to prepare the patient for the required, preferably gym-based, exercise program outlined below.

EXERCISE Begin with a private trainer for careful direction and education.

PATIENT EDUCATION AND MANAGEMENT (to be done during the initial one-on-one sessions and reinforced at all visits thereafter):

Instruct patients on **correct exercise technique**, including proper warm-up, breathing, joint protection, proper body positioning during the exercise, and how to cool-down and stretch afterwards.

Please work one muscle group at a time and perform extensive and extended **stretching** to each muscle group immediately after each one is exercised, before moving on to the next muscle group.

A careful interview should be performed at the start of each session to make apparent the effects, both good and bad, from the prior visit's therapy, and adjust therapy accordingly.

PROGRAM

Aerobic exercises are NOT allowed, not even low impact variety, until stamina improves.

Conditioning: work to improve strength and reverse the poor conditioning that results from Lyme, through a **whole-body** exercise program, consisting of light calisthenics and weight lifting, using small weights and many repetitions. This can be accomplished in exercise classes called "stretch and tone," or "body sculpture," or can be achieved with exercise machines, or carefully with free weights.

Each session should last one hour. If the patient is unable to continue for the whole hour, then modify the program to decrease the intensity to allow him/her to do so.

Exercise no more often than every other day. The patient may need to start by exercise every 4th or 5th day initially, and as his/her abilities improve, work out more often, but NEVER two days in a row. The days in between exercise sessions should be spent resting.

This **whole-body conditioning program** is what is required to achieve wellness. Simply placing the patient on a treadmill or an exercise bike is not acceptable (except briefly, as part of a warm-up), nor is a simple walking program.

PHYSICIAN'S SIGNATURE

MANAGING YEAST OVERGROWTH

Many patients with chronic illnesses including Lyme Disease develop an overgrowth of yeast. A basic strategy to combat this is to eat a full container of sugar-free, non-fruit flavored yogurt that contains active cultures daily, and take acidophilus, two after each meal. Here are some other suggestions:

MOUTH: Yeast problems usually begin in the mouth, for when thrush is present, organisms may repeatedly pass down into the GI tract where they cause the most problems. A tongue with a beige coating, bad breath, and a bad taste in the mouth are signs of oral yeast. Patients should use a toothpaste that contains surfactants (detergent-like cleaning agents), and antiseptic mouthwashes (Scope, Listerine, etc.), and brush the teeth, tongue, gums, cheeks and the roof of the mouth while holding the mouthwash in the mouth.

The most effective treatment, employed as a last resort, consists of using "Dakin's Solution" as a mouth rinse. This is a mixture of household liquid bleach (Clorox), one teaspoon in four ounces of water. A small amount is held in the mouth while brushing, then spit out, and repeated until the thrush has cleared. This is usually a one-time treatment, but may have to be repeated every few weeks.

After using an antiseptic to clean the mouth, it is necessary to immediately eat yogurt or chew an acidophilus capsule to replenish the beneficial flora in the mouth. Because the germ count after such a cleaning will be artificially reduced, and because yeasts are opportunists, they would be the first to come back. By having the yogurt or acidophilus then, a more normal oral flora will result and thrush will be better controlled.

Since yeast germs feed on sugars and starches, avoid simple carbohydrates including sugars, starches, and some fruits. Refer to the diet outlined below.

Prescription medications may be necessary. Mycelex troches and Nystatin liquid are not the best choice, for they contain large amounts of simple sugars. Instead, Nystatin oral powder is preferred, as it does not contain sugar. It is mixed with water, and swished and swallowed four times daily. Systemic antifungals tablets (Diflucan, Lamisil, Nizoral) may be necessary.

INTESTINAL TRACT: An overgrowth of yeast here will ferment dietary sugars and starches, forming acids, gas, and alcohols. Symptoms include gas, heartburn and/or pain in the stomach area, and because of the alcohol, there can be headaches, dizziness, lightheadedness, wooziness and post-meal fatigue. To clear intestinal yeast, first the oral cavity must be cleared so yeast does not reenter the system with every swallow. Avoid sweets, starches, fruits and juices to starve the germs. Use PLAIN yogurt daily, and acidophilus, 2 capsules three times daily after meals. Systemic antifungal medications may be needed.

VAGINAL: An occasional vaginal yeast infection can be controlled with products such as Monistat cream or suppositories. If it is a recurrent or ongoing problem, then it often reflects a simultaneous intestinal infection, re-infecting the genital area with every bowel movement. Therefore follow the above protocol for intestinal overgrowth, and use topical preparations such as Monistat concurrently for up to two weeks.

YEAST CONTROL DIET (Restricted carbohydrate regimen)
FOODS ALLOWED
Meat, fish, fowl, cheese, eggs, dairy, tofu

FRUITS
- **Only high fiber fruits are allowed**
- **Fruits are only allowed at the end of a meal, and never on an empty stomach**

ALLOWED

Grapefruit, tomatoes, avocado, lemons, limes

SMALL AMOUNTS ONLY! (The high fiber content in these makes up for the carbohydrates)

Pears, apples, strawberries, etc.

NOT ALLOWED

Oranges, watermelons, bananas, grapes, etc. (too much sugar and not enough fiber)

VEGETABLES
Green vegetables and salads are O.K. Avoid starchy vegetables (potato, rice, beans, etc.)

STARCHES
If it is made from flour, it is not allowed! (No breads, cereals, cake, etc.)

SWEETENERS
NOT ALLOWED

No sugars at all; no fructose or corn syrup, and no honey

ALLOWED (if tolerated)

Aspartame, Nutrasweet, Equal; saccharin products allowed but not recommended

DRINKS
ALLOWED

Vegetable juices, water, seltzer, diet sodas, coffee and tea without sugar or caffeine NOT ALLOWED Fruit juices, regular sodas, any drinks sweetened with sugars, syrups or honey

PATIENT INSTRUCTIONS ON BITE PREVENTION AND TICK REMOVAL
HOW TO PROTECT YOURSELF FROM TICK BITES
PROPERTY
Remove wood piles, rock walls, and bird feeders as these attract tick-carrying small animals and can increase the risk of acquiring Lyme.

INSECTICIDES: Property should be treated with a product called "Damminix." This consists of cardboard tubes containing cotton balls that have been dipped in insecticide. These tubes are placed around the property in the wooded areas and below shrubs. Mice, which are a key link in the propagation of Lyme disease, find the cotton and bring it back to their burrows to be used as nesting material, with the result being a big decrease in the number of ticks in the area. Unfortunately, after two years tick populations may rise again as other small animals that do not gather cotton become hosts to the ticks. Therefore, Damminix alone is not sufficient. Use this product in conjunction with liquid or granular insecticides.

LIQUID & GRANULAR PESTICIDES: Products meant for widespread application such as permethrin and its derivatives are preferred. They are available as a liquid concentrate and as granules. If liquid insecticides are used, application should be by fogging, not by coarse sprays. Apply these products in a strip a few feet wide at the perimeter of the lawn at any areas adjacent to woods and underbrush. Also treat any ornamental shrubs near the house that may serve as a habitat for small animals. The best time to apply these products is in late Spring and early Fall.

CLOTHING

When wearing long pants, tuck the cuffs into the socks so any ticks that get on shoes or socks will crawl on the outside of the pants and be less likely to bite. Also, light colored clothing should be worn so the ticks will be easier to spot. Smooth materials such as windbreakers are harder for ticks to grab onto and are preferable to knits, etc.

Tick repellents that contain "permethrin" (Permanone, Permakill) are meant to be sprayed onto clothing. Spray the clothes before they're put on, and let them dry first. Do not apply this chemical directly to the skin.

Ticks are very intolerant of being dried out. After being outdoors in an infested area, place clothes in the dryer for a few minutes to kill any ticks that may still be present.

SKIN

Insect repellents that contain "DEET" are somewhat effective when applied to the arms, legs, and around the neck. Do not use any repellent over wide areas of the body as they can be absorbed causing toxicity. Also, it is inadvisable to use a product that contains more than 50% DEET, and 25% concentrations are preferred. Use repellents cautiously on small children, as they are more susceptible to their toxic effects. Be aware that this repellent evaporates quickly and must be reapplied frequently.

Check carefully for ticks not only when home but frequently while still outside!

HOW TO REMOVE AN ATTACHED TICK

Using a tweezer (not fingers!), grasp the tick as close to the skin as possible and pull straight out. Then apply an antiseptic. Do not try to irritate them with heat or chemicals, or grasp them by the body, as this may cause the tick to inject **more** germs into your skin. Tape the tick to a card and record the date and location of the bite. Remember, the sooner the tick is removed, the less likely an infection will result.

APPENDIX
RATIONALE FOR TREATING TICK BITES

Prophylactic antibiotic treatment upon a known tick bite is recommended for those who fit the following categories:

> People at higher health risk bitten by an unknown type of tick or tick capable of transmitting Borrelia burgdorferi, e.g., pregnant women, babies and young children, people with serious health problems, and those who are immunodeficient.

> Persons bitten in an area highly endemic for Lyme Borreliosis by an unidentified tick or tick capable of transmitting B. burgdorferi.

> Persons bitten by a tick capable of transmitting B. burgdorferi, where the tick is engorged, or the attachment duration of the tick is greater than four hours, and/or the tick was improperly removed. This means when the body of the tick is squeezed upon removal, irri-

tated with toxic chemicals in an effort to get it to back out, or disrupted in such a way that its contents were allowed to contact the bite wound. Such practices increase the risk of disease transmission.

A patient, when bitten by a known tick, clearly requests oral prophylaxis and understands the risks. This is a case-by-case decision.

The physician cannot rely on a laboratory test or clinical finding at the time of the bite to definitely rule in or rule out Lyme Disease infection, so must use clinical judgment as to whether to use antibiotic prophylaxis. Testing the tick itself for the presence of the spirochete, even with PCR technology, is not reliable enough to guide your decision to treat, as false positives and false negatives occur.

An established infection by B. burgdorferi can have serious, long-standing or permanent, and painful medical consequences, and be expensive to treat. Since the likelihood of harm arising from prophylactically applied spirochetal antibiotics is low, and since treatment is inexpensive and painless, it follows that the risk benefit ratio favors tick bite prophylaxis.

EPILOGUE

After two years, we are still without a resolution. Still pinching pennies for groceries and medications. Why? The military has decided that anything and everything is more important than righting this wrong. Do we still complain? You bet. Do we still offer yet even more documentation of their illegal actions? Affirmative. Do we find anyone within the U.S. Army who will listen? Not on your life.

The U.S. Army at the Pentagon have assured me that they have received the documentation. They also stated that they are waiting (over 18 months now) for "other agencies and commands to respond." I would like to offer that if the "other agencies" and "other commands" are not responding to the Pentagon's request for information...they apparently have nothing to say!

The U.S. Army admit that they have more important issues at hand. A colonel I recently spoke with stated that the U.S. Army is concerned that they do not have enough soldiers at the present time. I would like to suggest that if the way they have treated this career soldier is any indication of their "Army of One" and their proud display of the Army Values, maybe time would be better spent on aligning the statements with the actions.

Until this military-created bollix is straightened out (and God only knows when that will be), we will stand firm in what my husband did was the legal and ethical way to handle the situation.

Until this blunder is cleared up, we remain in a state of limbo. We are without earned retirement, benefits, and Tim's belongings are still in South Korea. Pleas, requests, demands and even logic backed up with valid documentation has not budged the greensuiters off their cushy seats.

Could it be that we need an "act of congress" to encourage them to respond? We have contacted and have the assistance of two Congressmen. The Army continues to stall them...same as they impede us from having a normal life.

Still waiting for truth, justice, and the American way here. Is this why we served?

Visit Author Sue Vogan's Website and Find Out About The Radio Show She Hosts: "In Short Order" www.SueVogan.com

To Buy More Lyme-Related Books, DVDs, and Resources, visit www.LymeBook.com

www.ingramcontent.com/pod-product-compliance
Lightning Source LLC
Chambersburg PA
CBHW030919180526
45163CB00002B/402